Education and Support for Parenting

For Baillière Tindall:

Publishing Manager, Health Professions: Inta Ozols
Project Manager: Jane Dingwall
Design Direction: Judith Wright

Education and Support for Parenting

A Guide for Health Professionals

Edited by

Mary L. Nolan PhD MA BA (Hons) RGN
Antenatal Teacher/Tutor
The National Childbirth Trust
UK

Foreword by

Elisabeth Buggins MHSM DipHSM
Chairman
Walsall Community Health NHS Trust
West Midlands, UK

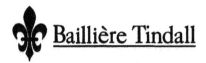
Baillière Tindall

EDINBURGH LONDON NEW YORK PHILADELPHIA ST LOUIS SYDNEY TORONTO 2002

BAILLIÈRE TINDALL
An imprint of Harcourt Publishers Limited

© Harcourt Publishers Limited 2002

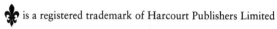 is a registered trademark of Harcourt Publishers Limited

The right of Mary Nolan to be identified as editor of this work has been asserted by her in accordance with the Copyright, Designs and Patents Act 1988

First published 2002

ISBN 0 7020 2641 7

British Library Cataloguing in Publication Data
A catalogue record for this book is available from the British Library

Library of Congress Cataloging in Publication Data
A catalog record for this book is available from the Library of Congress

Note
Medical knowledge is constantly changing. As new information becomes available, changes in treatment, procedures, equipment and the use of drugs become necessary. The editor, contributors and the publishers have taken care to ensure that the information given in this text is accurate and up to date. However, readers are strongly advised to confirm that the information, especially with regard to drug usage, complies with the latest legislation and standards of practice.

Transferred to Digital Print 2009

Printed and bound in the United Kingdom

The
publisher's
policy is to use
**paper manufactured
from sustainable forests**

Contents

Contributors

Caroline Archer BSc
Author, Independent Family Mentor/Consultant and Trainer for Adoption UK, West Glamorgan, UK

Caroline Archer is a long-standing member of Adoption UK (formerly PPIAS). She has four adopted children. Her experiences of raising several challenging children led her to explore the impact of very early experiences on the behaviour of adopted youngsters, both in psychological and neurophysiological terms. Caroline has recently begun collaborating with Family Futures Consortium, an independent attachment-based therapeutic consultancy. She is also establishing her own developmentally based attachment counselling and support service for adoptive families, known as Holding Families Together.

Alex Clark BSc
Assistant Psychologist, Special Parenting Service, Truro, Cornwall, UK

Alex Clark is an assistant psychologist with the Special Parenting Service. He gained a BSc Psychology degree at the University of Sheffield. Since graduating in 1998, Alex has worked with populations of autistic adults and children as well as with patients suffering from neuropsychological difficulties. He currently provides parenting and psychometric assessment, family support and home-based teaching programmes to learning-disabled parents throughout Cornwall.

Frances Hudson MA MEd BA (Hons) DipCouns
Freelance Trainer, Sex Educator and Counsellor; Member of the Independent Advisory Group to the Government's Teenage Pregnancy Unit

Frances Hudson worked for 20 years with very young mothers and their babies/toddlers at the Unit for Schoolgirl Mothers, Bristol, UK. Since retiring as head teacher there in 1994 she works as researcher, counsellor, trainer and tutor (school, FE college, HE, secure unit, Family Centre, Brook, PCTs) in the areas of effective communication skills, relationships and sexual health, and social work. All her work is informed by her awareness of the needs of children and young people, the influence of the family and 'good enough' parenting. She has twin daughters who have taught her a great deal.

Denise Marshall BA (Hons) Certificate in Massage, Anatomy and Physiology
National Childbirth Trust Antenatal Teacher; Lecturer, Holloway Prison, London, UK

Denise currently works with pregnant women and mothers and babies at Holloway Prison. She is also involved in community postnatal projects and teaches baby massage. Previously, Denise has taught antenatal classes for the National Childbirth Trust and worked in welfare rights and housing. Denise lives in London with her husband, Calum, and three children, Danny, Jake and Carmela.

Sue McGaw PhD MSc BA (Hons)
Chartered Consultant Clinical Psychologist/Head of Special Parenting Service, Truro, Cornwall, UK

Sue McGaw is a chartered consultant clinical psychologist for Cornwall Healthcare Trust. Her clinical experience spans 18 years of child psychiatry and learning disabilities. She is Head of the Special Parenting Service, which she founded in 1988, for parents with learning disabilities. She is also regarded as a leading expert in this field and is the British Psychological Society's spokesperson on this topic.

Olivia Montuschi BEd DipCouns
Freelance Consultant; Trainer; Writer, London, UK

Olivia Montuschi trained in the 1980s as a parent group facilitator with Exploring Parenthood and went on to develop and run courses for parents and professionals. She co-wrote Getting Connected, a first-step parenting programme, Parents Against Crime and Parenting Perspectives: a guide to teaching parenting skills. In 1995, she helped start the consultancy Parenting Connections, stepping down in 2000 to devote more time to writing and to the Donor Conception Network, a charity for parents of children conceived with the help of donated gametes. Olivia has two sons and a daughter.

Mary Nolan PhD MA BA (Hons) RGN
National Childbirth Trust Antenatal Teacher and Tutor; Trainer; Writer, Birmingham, UK

Mary Nolan trained as a nurse in the 1980s and then moved into antenatal education. She has been teaching pregnant and new parents for 14 years and during this time has written extensively for both parents and health professionals on pregnancy, birth, early parenting and adoptive parenting. She has three teenage daughters and lives in Worcestershire with her husband, Peter.

Judith Ockenden BSc (Hons) DipHE(Antenatal Teaching)
National Childbirth Trust Antenatal Teacher; Freelance Writer and Editor, Shropshire, UK

Judith Ockenden is now dedicated to her 'second career' in childbirth education, having worked for many years in medical/biological science publishing. In her NCT antenatal classes, preparation for parenthood is given equal weight with preparation for birth. She has published several articles on pregnancy, childbirth and parenting and is Chair of Shropshire Maternity Services Liaison Committee. Judith lives in Shropshire with her husband, Bob, and four daughters.

Nina Smith BA (Hons) MA
Antenatal Teacher/Tutor; Diploma in HE Development Coordinator at the
National Childbirth Trust, London, UK

Nina Smith has been an antenatal teacher for the National Childbirth Trust
since 1984 and has tutored antenatal teacher students since 1993. She co-led
the team which put together the NCT's university-validated Diploma of
Higher Education, Antenatal Education, and is currently the programme's
development coordinator. In 1998, she gained an MA by research, looking at
the role antenatal classes play for men in the transition to fatherhood. She is
also involved in an antenatal education project in Bosnia and Herzegovina
on behalf of UNICEF.

Elaine Spink MSc BA (Hons) PGCE DipHE(Antenatal Education)
Senior Lecturer in Primary Science Education, Manchester Metropolitan
University, Manchester, UK

Elaine Spink has been a lecturer in higher education for 10 years. Prior to that,
she was a primary school teacher and an advisory teacher for science. She has a
particular interest in active learning and has worked with the British Council,
providing active learning workshops for teachers in Indonesia, and written curriculum support materials for publishers. She is an antenatal teacher for the
National Childbirth Trust.

Debbie Valentine BA (Hons)
Deputy Head of Special Parenting Service, Truro, Cornwall, UK

Debbie Valentine graduated from the University of Florida, USA, with a BA
degree in Sociology. She has extensive experience working with families, providing assessments, interventions (individual and group), advocacy and support
in both the US and UK. Her primary focus is on empowering families to provide 'adequate' parenting and enhancing and promoting family preservation.
Debbie currently provides services for parents with mild to borderline learning
disabilities and assists the Head of the Special Parenting Service with programme development, monitoring and evaluation.

Sue White BA (Open) CertEd
Consultant and Trainer (Early Years, Disability), Kenilworth, Warwickshire, UK

After qualifying to teach the Early Years, Sue White taught child development
to advanced level students. Following this, she was the head of two nurseries
and then moved into the voluntary sector, developing services for children with
disabilities. She set up a Portage service and, in partnership with parents, developed a successful Family Centre over a 10-year period. Now working as a
Consultant, she has acted as manager for a SureStart Trailblazer programme,
and coordinated the Children's Fund delivery plan for Birmingham.

Foreword

Parenting is, as many have noted, the most important and challenging role undertaken by the majority of adults. Moss Kanter has described effective change management as less about the bold strike than the long march that follows it. If conception is the bold strike, parenting must be the long march!

Theories have abounded over the generations about how best to discharge the responsibilities the long march brings, together with dire warnings for those 'feckless' enough to ignore them. The concept of professional and social support for parents has only recently been articulated and incorporated into policy.

Over the past 25 years I have worked with the NHS as a senior manager, a parent of children with disabilities, a voluntary sector representative and an NHS trust chairman. During that time, NHS policy has changed from doing things *to* people, through doing things *for* them, to doing things *with* them. This shift has resulted from a fundamental recognition that providing sound information and fostering autonomy result in better physical outcomes and improved mental well-being. Engagement and building confidence have been found to be well worthwhile.

As a chairman in the NHS, I am very aware of the cultural and service changes both government and many staff would like to see. The NHS Plan (July 2000) states that 'The NHS has to be redesigned around the needs of the patient' and ' . . . a system designed around patients is a system with more power for patients'. This power will be based on:

■ a constructive relationship with healthcare providers
■ access to evidence-based, timely, relevant information
■ the availability of an advocate to assist the public in obtaining the information, advice and support they need.

Fine aspirations, but challenging to deliver in practice! This book is about how to incorporate these ideals into relationships between professionals and parents. I am aware that many staff in the statutory sector feel that they already embody them in their work. If so, this book will aid reflection and help refine practice. Others are aware that the systems within which they work fall short of the ideal but are unsure how to move from the certainties of being in control to the uncertainties of shared decision making. If you are one of these, this book will give you comfort in working through your anxieties, and practical help.

As a parent, I have borne and brought up four children, three of whom have serious, life-long medical conditions. My needs as a parent have been many but there are six things that have enabled me to confront and persevere through difficult reality.

1. *Respect* from friends and colleagues in both the statutory and voluntary sectors for the way I cope and interest in me as a person, not just as a mother.

2. *Positive reinforcement* – I think I have been luckier than many parents because my frequent contact with health professionals has given me lots of feedback about my parenting skills.
3. *Autonomy and choice* – these have been essential for my self-esteem. Parents of children with disabilities can find it very difficult to identify their role when there are so many instructions to follow and appointments to keep, with so many experts who seem to know more about the needs of their child than they do themselves.
4. *Time to talk and someone to listen* – the best people to listen have often been parents in a similar situation to my own.
5. *Information* – when I asked for it and when the active listening of others told them I needed it.
6. *Support* from someone who knew 'the system' and was available to advise me when needed.

These things have been of inestimable value to my children and me and I am eternally grateful to the professionals and voluntary workers who have provided them.

Much of the thinking articulated in this book develops the six themes I have outlined above and cites more objective evidence. It is about the powerful, constructive synergy between education and support. Whether you are a professional whose work is primarily to do with parents or someone who regularly meets parents as part of their working lives, it aims to provide you with inspiration and practical advice.

I hope this book will be widely read by workers involved in informing and supporting parents, in all their varied circumstances and needs. I hope, too, that reflecting on its messages will result in subtle but fundamental changes to working practices and relationships so that parents feel more confident in their important role and those working with them find greater satisfaction in enabling their potential.

Elisabeth Buggins
Walsall 2002

Preface

The quality of parenting is perhaps the single most important influence in shaping our society. Our sense of citizenship, of compassion and of belonging stems from the self-esteem, discipline and security that our parents foster in us. Being a parent in the 21st century is probably a more difficult task than it has ever been and yet expectations of parents have never been so high. Britain is not famed for its tolerance of children, especially young ones, and is quick to blame parents when their children misbehave. Parents have never had so many choices, but never have those choices been so difficult.

It is increasingly recognised by government, as it has long been by psychologists, that the quality of parenting in the early years sets the tone for the child's subsequent physical, emotional and educational development. One of government's recent flagship initiatives has been SureStart, now in its fifth wave. SureStart 'aims to improve the health and well-being of families and children before and from birth, so children are ready to thrive when they go to school' (DfEE 2000). It adopts a multidisciplinary strategy and a model of working in partnership with parents to support the parenting of children under the age of four.

The time is therefore ripe for a book which brings together the expertise of those who have been working in parent education for some time. There is no point in reinventing the wheel – much better to listen to what those with grassroots experience have to say and thereby identify best practice. The authors who have contributed to this book are experts in adult and parenting education. They are not ivory tower academics – each one has worked and still works with parents or specialises in supporting particular groups of parents.

Such specialist knowledge is both essential and hard to come by when working with groups of parents whose situation is different from what we might consider 'the norm'. This book looks at the needs of 'every' parent and also of a whole variety of 'special' parents. It asks and attempts to answer such questions as: How can women in prison be helped to make the transition to motherhood? What are the challenges facing parents who adopt a child? How does it feel to have carried, given birth to and parent a child whose genetic material is not your own? What are the most effective ways of communicating with parents who have learning difficulties? How can you help the parent of a child with a disability to celebrate the child rather than focus on the disability?

This book explores the skills that health professionals and allied workers need in order to support parents' efforts to be 'good enough'. It looks at the basic skills of adult education and how these can be applied in one-on-one interviews with parents and in parenting groups. It tries to identify some methods of evaluating the success of educational encounters with parents and of determining how to engage more effectively with parents in the future.

Educating parents goes hand in hand with supporting them and support is sometimes all that is required to build parents' confidence to *educate themselves*. This book talks a great deal about how to support parents and about parents supporting each other. It talks about weaning parents off dependence on professionals by enabling them to identify the information and skills they need and find support in applying them to their individual circumstances.

Above all, the book is firmly grounded in 'the real world'. It identifies the key issues for parents in varying circumstances *from their point of view* and so aims to transform a culture of advice giving into one of empathy and support. Health professionals have known for years that giving advice is rarely successful. By and large, adults do not like being advised. They listen politely and then ignore what has been said to them or cherry pick the pieces of advice they think useful, or aggressively reject the proffered 'help' because it is seen as irrelevant. This book is about empathising with parents so that the educational encounter becomes a means for them to identify for themselves what would be best in their situation. Parents may, of course, know what they should do, but still not do it. If they have been helped to identify a problem and a strategy for dealing with it and choose not to, the responsibility for the outcome lies firmly with them – which is where it should lie.

Each chapter in this book reflects the individual 'voice' of the author, and so the style varies from the formal to the far less formal. To assist readers in understanding and retaining ideas and information presented, figures, boxes and lists of Key Points have been used. In some chapters, you will find icons to indicate Activities ⬚ and Reflection Points ⬚.

The inspiration for the book stems from my own work with parents and a sense, which has grown stronger year by year, that parents need and deserve support in a world where their children have access to knowledge and opportunities which were certainly not available to them. My thanks must therefore go firstly to all the parents with whom I have come into contact over 15 years of teaching antenatal classes and supporting parents postnatally. Secondly, I want to thank those who have contributed to the book for the intelligent and committed effort each one made to understanding and supporting my vision and incorporating it into their chapters. My three daughters, on whom my personal parenting skills have been honed, also deserve mention for their not insignificant part in the evolution of this book!

Mary L Nolan

1   'Good-enough' parenting

Mary Nolan

INTRODUCTION

There are over 16 million families in Britain. Four-fifths of dependent children still live in a family with two parents and nine out of 10 of those parents are married. More than eight in 10 fathers still live with all their biological children and more than seven in 10 are doing so within their first family (Family Policy Studies Centre 2000).

PARENTS UNDER PRESSURE

These facts may seem to suggest that 'the family' in Britain today is not so very different from what it has been for centuries. Yet the Family Policy Studies Centre also informs us that family breakdown is currently costing the public purse about £5 billion a year and that the fastest growing group of parents is never-married, lone mothers. Annual marriage rates are at their lowest levels since records began 160 years ago and if present divorce rates continue, it is estimated that 28% of children will experience the divorce of their parents before they reach the age of 16. Clearly the family *is* changing and *is* under considerable pressure. Parents are being scrutinised as never before and appear to have become the latest scapegoat for the ills of society. Like schools, parents find themselves named and shamed if their offspring fail to become law-abiding citizens.

Government and health professionals, even in today's climate of scepticism and scandals, play a major role in formulating and consolidating society's beliefs about the duties and effectiveness of parents.

Since the days of Bowlby and Winnicott, society has considered that the relationship between parent and child, and especially between mother and child, is the ultimate arbiter of what kind of adult the child becomes. Such a simplification fails to acknowledge, first, the restrictions placed upon parents by adverse social circumstances and the disintegration of the extended family and local community, and second, the fact that the world in which today's children are growing up is light years away from the world in which their parents grew up. Technology is such that life in the year 2000 bears very little resemblance even to life in the 1970s. The choices facing young people and the opportunities available to them are infinitely more complex than those which their parents enjoyed.

The job of being a parent in the 21st century and of transmitting parenting skills to the next generation has probably never been so difficult. Fagot (1995) notes:

FIGURE 1.1

Guilty of being
a bad parent

THE MOTHER of a persistent truant yesterday became the first parent to face the full force of Jack Straw's new clampdown on unruly teenagers. Lena Summers will have to attend lessons herself on how to become a better parent. She was hauled before magistrates after her 14 year old son, David, missed 217 out of 256 days at school ..... She will be required to attend a three-month course of lessons to teach her how to curb her son's behaviour. And both of them could receive counselling ..... [The Home Secretary] borrowed the idea from the USA where it has been used effectively to supervise struggling parents and children. Simply fining parents has not worked in the past.

(front page: Daily Mail 13 July 2000)

Society is harsh in its judgement of those who fail in these domains [of parenting], yet dictionaries do not even define the word, and our society requires no special training for parenting. (p. 163)

Most parents are eager to do their best. Testimony to their search for information and guidance can be found by scanning the shelves of any bookstore. I recently came across the following titles pressed tightly together in a section of a city-centre bookshop dedicated to the art of parenting.

- *501 Ways to Be a Good Parent*
- *Raising a Child Responsibly in a Sexually Permissive World*
- *Head Start: How to Develop Your Child's Mind*
- *How to Increase your Child's Verbal Intelligence*
- *Self-Esteem for Boys*
- *Self-Esteem for Girls*
- *The Whole Parenting Guide – Strategies, Resources and Inspiring Stories for Holistic Parenting and Family Living*
- *Parachutes for Parents*
- *25 Stupid Mistakes Parents Make*

There is clearly a large market for such books, indicating a substantial need. I found the titles of the books fascinating – indicative of the multiple demands made of parents and the shame and guilt they feel, or are made to feel, should they make 'stupid mistakes'! Yet it is too easy to disregard the fact that parents' ability to perform their role 'is a function of the ratio of the demands made on them and resources available to them' (Henry 1996: 25). This book is about how health professionals can become active, useful and energising resources for parents.

DEBRIEFING PERSONAL EXPERIENCES

Any assessment of 'good-enough' parenting must be based on the needs of both children and parents. And anyone pronouncing on what constitutes 'good-enough' parenting must have taken the time and had the courage to revisit, reflect on and understand their own experiences of being parented. The baggage we carry around with us as a result of the years we spent being mothered and fathered is a heavy burden indeed. In terms of assisting parents to fulfil their roles more sensitively and effectively, the phrase 'Physician, heal thyself' could not be more appropriate. Our concept of what parents are, what they do, what they do not do and how they should behave is firmly rooted in our own experiences with our parents. Until this has been accepted, and understood, we are in no position to assess the parenting efforts of others.

Most training for people wishing to lead parent education courses is underpinned by careful debriefing of personal experiences of being parented. The National Childbirth Trust's Diploma Course in Antenatal Education includes a module on reflective practice with the following outline content.

- Impact of personal experiences of giving birth on early parenting.
- Impact of being parented on own parenting.
- Benefits of debriefing birth and parenting experiences.
- Negative effects of inadequate debriefing of birth and parenting experiences.
- Impact of birth and parenting experiences on motivation to become an antenatal teacher, attitudes towards maternity care, attitudes towards expectant parents.

Positive Parenting runs workshops for parent educators where reflection on issues such as the following is invited.

- Were you able to talk about your feelings to your parents?
- How was conflict managed when you were a child?
- How were you disciplined as a child?
- To what extent are you doing/did you do the same thing with your own children?

Elaine Spink's chapter on Supporting Adult Learning (Chapter 2) and Judith Ockenden's on Antenatal Education for Parenting (Chapter 5) look in some detail at the importance of debriefing.

WHAT CHILDREN NEED

The needs of children have probably never been so well understood as they are today. Research has continued apace since the 1950s and attracts some of the brightest and most committed social scientists, psychologists and educational-ists in academe. Theories of how best to parent have been advanced and debunked. At the start of the millennium, it is no longer the ultimate sin for mothers to go out to work – welcome reassurance for so many women. We know (and have known for some time but the tabloid press is often slow to abandon its prejudices) that it is not the *duration* of interaction between the mother and child that is significant but the *intensity* of that interaction (Rutter 1981). Another welcome volte face was the recognition by psychologists that it is all right to comfort crying babies. Ignoring the distress of infants in no way guarantees that they will grow into children who are self-controlled, consider-ate of others and self-denying! Babies who have learned that their parents do not respond when they are in distress are far more likely to become children who are clingy, lacking in confidence, unwilling to take the initiative and aggres-sive in their determination to get what they want (Ainsworth 1989). Henry (1996) describes the relationship between the caregiving and the attachment sequences in Figure 1.2.

FIGURE 1.2	*Caregiving and attachment (based on Henry 1996)*

Baby hungry ⟶ baby cries ⟶ mother feeds baby ⟶ baby satisfied ⟶ baby plays

Stress ⟶ demand ⟶ caregiving ⟶ assuagement ⟶ latitude

In a state of 'latitude', the baby feels confident, is alert and eager to engage with the outside world. What a relief for women brought up by mothers who parented in the 1950s and 1960s to find that they did not have to harden their hearts against their baby's distress for fear that picking him up would create a demanding and ultimately delinquent child! Yet puritanical attitudes are strangely resistant to change. Even today, in my antenatal classes, the debate about whether you should pick up a crying baby remains a lively one!

We know that infants need empathic parents who tune in to the signals they are sending, intuit their needs and respond accordingly. We know that they need emotional warmth and love, touching, rocking, holding and smiling. The mood of the mother following the birth of her child, the nature of the contact between them during the first 3 months of the baby's life and the attitude of the mother towards feeding her baby all predict the child's development, for example, in terms of his ability to understand and use language at the age of 3 (Bee et al 1982). We know that small children do not need to be primarily attached to their mothers, although for many, the mother is the primary focus of attach-ment. They can also become primarily attached to their fathers or other carers.

Babies need feeding, attention to their basic physical needs and protection from harm. A mother's ability to meet these needs will depend on her own men-tal health. Brockington (1996) explains in detail how postnatal unhappiness and depression have long-lasting effects on the physical, social and mental well-being of the child. It therefore behoves health professionals whose concern is with the neonatal period to assist the pregnant or new mother in identifying sources of support. McIntosh (1993) reports that 'Mothers who were relatively unsupported in the early stages of motherhood were more likely to become depressed than those with a more supportive network' (p. 248). Intervention studies (Clement 1995, Oakley et al 1996) have shown that social support offered by health professionals during pregnancy must extend into the postnatal period to ensure continuity of caregiving during the critical period after birth when women are especially vulnerable. Extending 'listening visits' into the postnatal period enables midwives and health visitors to detect the early signs of mental illness and arrange for prompt referral. Babies need mothers or primary caregivers who are mentally robust.

Children need to play because through play, they explore the world, learn what is safe and what is not and start to develop an understanding of their own powers and limitations. Adults are responsible for the environment of play in which the toddler finds himself. They provide the range of toys available to him; they set the limits to his freedom and they determine the level of ambient stimulation.

Through communication with adults and older children, small children acquire language. The speed with which language is acquired and the range of verbal tools available to the child are entirely dependent on the amount of time older people spend talking to him. Children do not develop their language skills by playing with children of the same age (although they may develop other skills). Language skills can, however, be assisted by older children and an environment which includes children of different ages (such as the preschool playground) is a rich one.

The task of babyhood is to develop trust and this is acquired in direct proportion to the responsiveness and empathy of the adults caring for him. The tasks of toddlerhood are to develop autonomy and initiative. Autonomy is a function of the extent to which small children are helped to help themselves, to make appropriate choices and to understand the causes of conflict and how to resolve it.

BOX 1.1	*Developing autonomy in toddlers*
	Henry (1996) describes tactics adopted by caregivers at a nursery in Australia:
	Encouraging self-help by permitting toddlers many small choices that were genuinely theirs to make: which of the two shirts in their bag they would put on, whether to eat the banana next or the sandwich. Successful choices that built feelings of confidence and mastery reduced the need to be negative. (p. 22)

The task of developing initiative is a function of the child's growing understanding of what people do and what the consequences of those actions are. It is assisted by being with people, watching them and interacting with them.

The child's need to watch makes the modelling of behaviour by adults a key issue. It is insufficient for the child to receive warmth and comfort from a caregiver if he does not see the same warmth and comfort giving in evidence between his mother and his father or between his principal caregivers. The relationships between the mother and child, between the father and child and between the mother and father are equal in their influence on the child's development of trust, autonomy and initiative.

BOX 1.2	*Children's needs*

Mortley's very useful discussion (1998: 7–10) of concepts of 'good-enough' parenting lists children's needs as follows.

- *Basic physical care* – warmth, shelter, food, rest, hygiene, protection from danger
- *Affection* – holding, cuddling, kissing, admiration, patience, time
- *Security* – continuity of care and a predictable environment
- *Stimulation of innate potential* – by praise and responsiveness to questions and play
- *Guidance and control* – which includes discipline within the child's understanding and a model for the child to copy
- *Responsibility* – giving the child responsibility for small things and allowing him to gain experience through mistakes as well as successes
- *Independence* – allowing him to make his own decisions

In middle childhood, parents spend less time with their children and outside influences become stronger. Collins et al (1995) note that this decline in time together is relatively greater for parents with lower levels of education. Discipline becomes a key issue and the need continues for this to be exercised by parents and caregivers who model the behaviour that is being required of the child. The environment cannot be too punitive or children lose their self-esteem and confidence and are unwilling to explore their environment further for fear of making mistakes ending in retribution. Maccoby (1984) considers that appropriate discipline is far better based on an appeal to the child's sense of fairness or to the need to return favours or reminders of the parents' greater knowledge than the threat of punishment or the promise of rewards. While it is clearly important to discourage antisocial behaviour, discipline must be related to the child's understanding of what is personally or socially acceptable and to their need to push the boundaries and discover for themselves what is safe and what is not. The dictum that parents should say 'yes' at least nine times for every once they say 'no' is probably a sound one.

Parents nurture the physical, emotional and spiritual well-being of their school-age children by means of effective discipline, sensitivity to their psychological state, solving problems as they arise and providing positive reinforcement of desirable behaviour. Discipline, problem solving and positive reinforcement depend on *monitoring* which is related to Bornstein's concept of *empathy* (1995) and Henry's notion of *responsiveness* (1996). Parents' ability to monitor children's personal, social and spiritual development depends on their ability to put themselves in their children's shoes and parents' ability to solve problems depends on their empathy with their child's difficulties. Positive reinforcement necessitates a fine balance between encouraging behaviour and attitudes that are socially and personally responsible and discouraging inappropriate ones in such a way as to preserve the child's self-esteem and eagerness to explore the world and test out his capacities.

Collins et al (1995) state that the quality of parenting in the middle years of childhood reflects and is rooted in the relationship patterns established in the preschool years. Therefore, fostering and advancing the empathy between parents and their babies and toddlers will assist in the development and application of positive parenting skills later on. It is for this reason that much of the present book looks at how to facilitate learning about parenting in the antenatal period and during the early years of childhood.

WHAT PARENTS NEED

It is, of course, true to say that most of the business of learning about what parenting means and how it is carried out is undertaken while parents are themselves children. Those who seek to provide parenting education for any group of clients must do so in the full knowledge that the parenting blackboard is written over with a multitude of scripts by the time the parents present themselves in a surgery, in court or on a parenting course. Grimshaw & McGuire's research (1998) into what parents want from parenting programmes suggests that many are aware of the need to break the mould of parenting set in their own childhood. One parent is quoted as follows.

I couldn't see anything else probably, because that was in my childhood, too . . . My father was violent towards us, as far as I can remember, and I feel that I was actually following a lot in his footsteps.

Many parents have said similar things to me in antenatal classes.

I suppose in many ways I had an excellent upbringing – I didn't want for anything. My parents were loving and allowed me to have some freedom even though I was an only child and that must have been difficult for them. But they also had the knack of making me feel guilty about things that they really didn't want me to do and I think they were quite puritanical because they always seemed to be critical of me having a good time! I think I've been far too critical of my own children as a result, although I try not to be. (Leanne, aged 29)

Unlearning the lessons of childhood is a fundamental component of parenting programmes and assisting parents to reflect on where certain patterns of parenting behaviour come from is essential in any approach, structured or unstructured, formal or informal, to parenting education.

Knowledge and freedom from misconceptions

Parents need knowledge and to be freed from misconceptions. For example, they need to know that you cannot spoil babies. So many parents are haunted by the fear that if they spare the rod, they will spoil the child. This is a dictum that was, in the past, reinforced by wrong advice on the feeding of babies which meant that more than one generation of mothers sat with their hands over their ears, trying to ignore their babies' desperate crying, because they had been told that feeding must be by the clock. We now know that the physiology of breast-feeding is fundamentally hostile to clock watching. Bottlefeeding also works best if led by the demands of the baby rather than by the will of the parents. The dangers of apathy also need to be recognised. Babies are far more likely to be emotionally damaged by lack of response from their parents than by too eager a response.

This is the sort of information that, when delivered by a health professional with the authority that his or her role carries, can transform parents' relationship with their baby or child. Conveying to the parents of a child of any age who is extremely demanding that the outcomes of parenting are not entirely dependent upon the actions and attitudes of parents but depend in part on the personality of the child being parented is also immensely reassuring. What happens in the womb during pregnancy and what happens during the birth mould the child in ways that are generally totally beyond the ability of parents to control. The child is born with the beginnings of a personality that may prove difficult or even intransigent, regardless of the parents' best efforts.

> Psychological stress during pregnancy may predispose the child to react in an undesirable way to subsequent adverse environments and so predispose him to behaviour problems, including juvenile delinquency. Preterm delivery has been found in controlled studies to be associated with behaviour problems at school age, especially with defective concentration and attention deficit disorders. (Illingworth 1991:211)

It is important for all health professionals who encounter parents, whether in the arena of parenting education, healthcare or counselling, to recognise and enable parents to recognise that there are different ways of interacting with infants and children. It has been argued in the past that maternal behaviour is (or should be) a consistent phenomenon, irrespective of the nature of the interaction with the child, the time at which the interaction takes place or its context (Winnicott 1957). Yet it is quite clear that the nature of the engagement with the child will and should vary if the child is to learn that adults have different moods and levels of energy, just as he does himself.

Mothers (and fathers) engage in a wide range of activities, all of which could be described as 'good-enough' parenting. Some mothers like face-to-face play with their children; others prefer reading to their child; some will talk to their children whatever they are doing, throughout the day, and others will have periods of intense verbal exchange with their child, followed by periods of quiet. Children often seek to engage their mothers in play while fathers frequently initiate sessions of rowdy horseplay which are adored by their children precisely because of their spontaneity. The variety of caregiving practices demonstrated by the different carers with whom a child is placed, and the different kinds of play in which various adults engage him, form a rich texture of learning opportunities. There is no single right way of giving care to a child or of playing or interacting with him.

Receiving up-to-date information about the effects on children of mothers going out to work is important for working women, lessening the burden of guilt that so many seem to carry around with them. The advantages of working include not only the financial rewards but also an increase in women's confidence and self-esteem and a decreased incidence of depression. The needs of parents for independence as well as companionship and the satisfaction of stretching themselves intellectually deserve recognition. Perhaps these needs have never been so pressing as they are now when parenting is often a very lonely experience. It is accepted that mothering does not have to be provided by one person only and that the tasks of mothering, both emotional and physical, can be shared between a number of responsive adults, of either gender, while the child remains principally attached to his mother (Rutter 1981).

Acceptance and approval

Bearing in mind that a wide range of parenting styles will successfully nurture the physical and emotional well-being of children and that a wide range of care-givers can provide the warmth and stimulation necessary for the child's development, acceptance of most parenting practices (excluding those demonstrably harmful) is usually appropriate. Acceptance and approval need to be communicated to parents, as parents receive many brickbats but very few bouquets for their efforts. Caroline Flint talks movingly in *Sensitive Midwifery* (1986) about how the new mother's confidence is affected by comments on the way in which she is feeding her baby. The vulnerability of women in relation to criticism of the food they give to their families should never be underestimated. After all, the prime task of mothering is to ensure that the children are adequately fed. To tell a new mother that her baby is putting on too much or too little weight, that she should be breastfeeding if she is bottlefeeding or bottlefeeding if she is breastfeeding is profoundly undermining. If her feeding technique is inappropriate, this needs discussing with her in such a way that, first and foremost, her efforts to be a good-enough mother are acknowledged and only then are ways in which she could do even better suggested.

Pugh & De'Ath (1984:17–19) argue that what parents need in order to be 'good enough' is:

- information and knowledge about children's health
- information and knowledge about what to expect at different stages of child development
- parenting skills to respond and adapt to changing needs and demands
- understanding of themselves as parents and as people.

Nurturing relationships

Bornstein (1995) contends that mothers require supportive relationships with 'secondary parents' who are defined as husbands, lovers or grandparents. After mothers and fathers, grandparents are the single most important source of preschool childcare (Family Policy Studies Centre 2000). There is evidence to suggest that mothers who are supported by figures who are able to parent their children in case of need, and nurture the mothers as well, are more able to respond sensitively to their infants than women who do not enjoy such relationships (Parke et al 1992). A mother who is supported by a health professional whom she meets regularly and who is able to model good-enough parenting with her children, as well as encouraging, reassuring and building her self-esteem, might find in this relationship the 'secondary parent' whom she needs. At a time when the fastest growing group of parents is single, never-married lone mothers (Family Policy Studies Centre 2000), many women will turn to health professionals or volunteers as secondary parents in the absence of the people who usually fill that role.

Empowerment

A woman's first pregnancy involves the critical transition from being the daughter of a mother to becoming the mother of a child. It is a period of intense vulnerability as well as a unique learning opportunity. The process of building her confidence in her ability to be a good-enough parent must start at this point. Yet everything conspires against the empowerment of the mother-to-be. She is prevented from forming an immediate relationship with her unborn child by a barrage of antenatal tests which require her to confront the possibility that she might terminate the pregnancy almost as soon as she has found out it exists. Women who opt for a mid-term amniocentesis must wait a minimum of 10 days (sometimes, 2 or 3 weeks) before they find out whether their baby is normal. Many women will put their pregnancies 'on hold' during this period, distancing themselves emotionally from their child lest the child is never to be born. Even when the results of a test are good, the mother may not find her anxieties alleviated.

> [Midwife commenting] A lady came along and her AFP was slightly low and she had an amniocentesis and everything was fine. But it didn't reassure her; she spent the rest of her pregnancy worrying so, for her, it didn't work. (Quoted in Nolan 1997: xxvi)

As more and more antenatal tests capable of screening for or diagnosing abnormalities in the unborn child become available, the greater are the problems for health professionals and pregnant women. Antenatal testing should always be preceded by counselling to help the woman understand what kind of information the test is providing (an estimate of the likelihood of the baby being affected by a particular condition or a diagnosis of that condition) and what she might do given an unfavourable outcome. The time to provide such counselling is simply not available, with the result that I meet many women in antenatal classes who tell me that they know their baby has definitely not got Down's syndrome or any other major abnormality because their AFP test was OK! This undermines the rights of parents to make informed choices about their children and, in the event of a woman giving birth to a disabled infant, seriously compromises her relationship with that baby whom she had believed to be normal.

Building parents' confidence depends in pregnancy and childbirth (as it does during the whole parenting experience) on the quality of the communication which health professionals can demonstrate in their encounters with parents. Communication in relation to parenting has been the subject of a great deal of research and discussion in the literature. In 1983, Shapiro et al noted that the quality and the amount of information received by some parents were very poor.

> The lower the class of the patient [read 'parent'] the greater is likely to be her desire for information on a wide range of topics. The lower the class of the respondent, the less likely the respondent is to obtain information she wants. (p. 143)

And 10 years later, Fleissig (1993) wrote:

> Doctors and midwives have difficulty in communicating with single women and those belonging to ethnic minority groups. (p. 74)

At the turn of the millennium, a teenage mum writes about her time in hospital after the birth of her daughter.

> The hospital were no help at all. They treated me as if I was stupid and took it for granted that I wouldn't cope, but when I asked for help, they didn't want to know. (Hadley 2000:95)

Labour and birth form a critical part of the transition to parenthood when fostering the mother's sense of control and self-confidence is vital. I was recently at dinner with an obstetrician who declared that the notion that giving birth could be a peak experience in a woman's life was nonsense. I found his attitude difficult to credit when so much work has been done in the area of understanding women's needs during labour and how the kind of birth she has impacts on her relationship with her baby. Oakley's study (1980) of the relationship between what happens to a woman during childbirth and her postnatal mood suggests at a high level of significance that 'low control felt in labour' and 'dissatisfaction with birth management' are related to postnatal depression. Oakley also found that 'low self-image as mother' which resulted from a woman's perception that she had been out of control during labour was significantly related to poor feelings for her baby. Sosa et al (1980) and Kennell et al (1991) argue that it is essential to preserve a woman's self-esteem during childbirth by helping her to maximise her own resources for coping with pain, by praising her and by keeping her fully informed about and involved in decisions regarding pain relief, management of labour and the condition of her baby.

For some particularly vulnerable women, the experience of childbirth can make or break their relationship with their infant. Parratt (1994) discusses the needs of women who have suffered sexual abuse.

> In identifying the varying needs necessary for the survivors of incest to experience a positive birth experience, such as trust, continuity of care, privacy, security and knowledge, it has become clear from all the findings that control is the predominant need of all. (p. 38)

The need for parents, at whatever stage of the parenting continuum, to feel in control of decisions regarding the welfare of their children, and the detrimental impact on mental health when that decision-making responsibility is taken away, are clear. Health professionals, whatever their level of interaction with parents, should aim to convey information and offer support in such a way that parents' autonomy is preserved and enhanced. If I tell you my problem and you tell me what to do, I know that I am helpless. So the next time I have a problem, I do not even attempt to find a solution, I simply turn to you again. In this way, a cycle of dependence (Fig. 1.3) is perpetuated.

FIGURE 1.3   *Cycle of dependence*

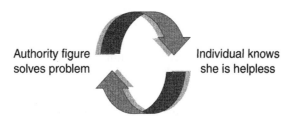

Authority figure
solves problem

Individual knows
she is helpless

RESOURCES

Gowen (1979) lists three kinds of resources that need to be available to parents to enable them to be 'good enough'.

1. *Internal resources* – childrearing skills, knowledge and attitudes, problem-solving skills, physical and mental health, intelligence
2. *Intra-household resources* – economic resources, models for good parenting, cooperative household helpers, supportive interpersonal relationships
3. *Extra-household (community) resources* – both formal (e.g. employment, educational, health, childcare) and informal (support from friends, relatives, neighbours)

Parenting education operates primarily as an 'internal resource' in facilitating the acquisition of childrearing and problem-solving skills, knowledge and self-awareness. By so doing, it will play its part in improving the physical and mental health of both parents and their children. Health professionals may also be able to offer some support in the area of extra-household resources and they can refer parents to organisations such as Home-Start, Newpin and the National Childbirth Trust which provide befriending services. Yet it should be acknowledged that parenting education and support cannot achieve their full potential if economic resources (intra-household resources) and access to many extra-household resources are severely curtailed.

Parenting cannot be placed on the educational agenda and parents then wiped off every other. Government must shoulder its responsibilities in the areas of economic and formal community resources if its commitment to better parenting is to bear fruit.

Conditions under which parenting appears to be particularly stressful have been identified by parents themselves as follows (based on Grimshaw & McGuire 1998).

- Parenting three children under the age of 5
- Parenting more than three children
- Problem behaviour in at least one child
- Health concerns about at least one child
- Parenting a disabled child
- Being a lone parent
- Being separated from a child
- Being a young mother
- Being a refugee
- Suffering from depression
- Having a health problem
- Having a housing problem
- Worries about money or work
- Unsupportive or abusive partner
- Little support from adult relatives
- Low household income.

However, parents do not need help all the time. There will be periods of turmoil followed by more stable periods when parents are in a position to provide help to others. In this book, Sue White (Chapter 4) discusses how partnerships can be established with experienced parents to enrich educational and support initiatives for less experienced or struggling parents.

PARENTING EDUCATION: WHEN AND HOW?

Grimshaw & McGuire (1998) noted that half the parents they surveyed wanted to access a parenting programme before their child reached the age of three. While the pressures of parenting teenagers are generally acknowledged to be considerable, so little work has been done in the area that parents tend not to ask for classes when their children are this age because they have not been available. Many of the parents in Grimshaw's study wished to be able to attend classes with their partners, although some were doubtful whether they would feel free to say what they really thought in the presence of the other person. This ties in with Nina Smith's research (Chapter 6) and her discussion of the difficulties of attracting fathers to parenting classes.

Various approaches to parenting education have been utilised. Pugh & De'Ath (1984) provide a useful definition of parenting education which would surely encompass all the most successful (because truly parent-centred) programmes.

> Parent education comprises a range of educational and supportive measures which help parents and prospective parents to understand their own social, emotional, psychological and physical needs and those of their children and enhances the relationship between them. It should be available to all parents and prospective parents. It is a lifelong process and as such will have a different emphasis at different stages of the life cycle. Its emphasis should be on individuals' roles and relationships in the here-and-now, as well as with their future roles and relationships. (p. 208)

Aims and learning outcomes for parenting programmes can be summarised as follows (Barlow & Stewart-Brown 2000).

Aims

To help parents develop:

■ appropriate expectations (of themselves and their children)
■ self-awareness and self-esteem
■ a positive approach to discipline
■ empathy.

Learning outcomes

Parents are able to:

■ use praise
■ understand their children's emotional needs
■ help their children express how they are feeling

- set clear boundaries
- maintain effective positive discipline/find alternatives to punishment.

Behavioural programmes, based on social learning theory, focus on children's behaviour and on understanding how acceptable behaviour can be cultivated and unacceptable discouraged. Such programmes often include problem-solving and management skills. Humanistic programmes are more varied and focus on how parents communicate with their children and how conflicts can be resolved by active listening on the part of parents. Parents are helped to examine the way in which they think about their children and their children's behaviour and to examine their feelings in the context of how they themselves were parented. Other groups which do not fall directly under the 'behavioural' or 'humanistic' umbrellas are principally discussion groups, often led by parents themselves, where problems are shared and experiences pooled so that successful parenting practices can be passed from one parent to another.

Pugh & De'Ath (1984) warn of the dangers of prescriptive programmes of parenting education, which imply that there is only one way of managing children's behaviour or one approach to successful parenting. This is to ignore the complexity of parenting and the fact that each parent's personal history, socioeconomic circumstances, beliefs and attitudes and each of their children are very different. It is, therefore, far more appropriate to base parenting programmes on principles rather than on prescriptions. Advice is rarely well received by parents and even when it is, Grimshaw & McGuire (1998) remind us that it will be diluted by parents in their attempt to adapt it to their particular circumstances. Parents do not welcome generalisations which have no immediate relevance to their particular children or their particular circumstances. For this reason, successful parenting courses are often those which have been designed as a result of extensive consultation with parents from the targeted group or area (see Sue White, Chapter 4) or which are run by parents themselves. Organisations such as Parent Network invite parents who have attended a course to consider training as facilitators themselves, so that courses reflect both what parents want to learn and how they want to learn it.

Barlow & Stewart-Brown's survey (2000) summarises the ways in which parents benefited from taking part in parenting programmes. What parents most appreciated was the support they gained from being in a group with other parents and the opportunity to be themselves in an accepting environment. The realisation that their difficulties were not peculiar to them was both reassuring and empowering. Once parents realised that they shared many concerns, they were able to move towards common solutions. Parents were wary of being 'taught' how to be a parent, preferring a facilitator who supported them rather than telling them what they should do. However, feedback from group leaders was accepted when presented as observations and suggestions rather than as advice. As a result of attending a parenting course, many parents felt less guilty about their parenting and were better able to understand that they had rights and feelings, too, as well as their children!

> It made me recognise that I was a human being as well, you know. And I have needs and requirements as well whereas before I was trying to be the super-duper wonderful parent, trying to do everything without actually paying any attention to myself. (Quoted in Barlow & Stewart-Brown 2000:13)

Those who engage in parenting education need to be:

- empathic and warm
- respectful and encouraging
- non-critical
- flexible
- able to see the funny side of things
- enthusiastic
- happy in the role of non-expert (Barlow & Stewart-Brown 2000)

Health professionals may have to work hard to convince parents that it is their (the parents') agenda that is paramount at the classes. Even when they are keen to encourage parents to devise strategies for coping with their own problems, they may be thwarted by parents who persist in seeing them as authority figures and problem solvers and who ask: 'But tell me what you would do in my situation'. The temptation to provide ready-made solutions not tailored to individual circumstances, and therefore unlikely to work, can be considerable. Yet ultimately, the failure to empathise with parents so that the problem can be addressed on their terms and using their resources undermines parents' confidence in their own abilities to parent their children.

Thoughtful practical arrangements are essential for running a successful parenting programme.

BOX 1.3	*Practical arrangements for parenting courses*

Venue
- A location close to the parents whom it is hoped will attend.

Cost
- Free or perhaps a nominal sum payable on a weekly basis (people are inclined to value more highly something they have to pay for).

Crèche
- Perhaps run by parents who have previously attended the course (it is children who prevent parents from attending a parenting programme!).

There are many ways in which parenting education can be delivered. Health professionals will frequently find themselves in one-to-one situations with parents where parenting is the overt reason for the consultation or forms part of the problem being presented. They may provide monthly lectures at the surgery on specific topics, during which information can be given and discussion encouraged. Informal groups for parents and small children can be set up at the local health centre with a health visitor or practice nurse available to answer questions, although the primary aim is for parents to support each other by sharing problems and coping strategies. A parent might be invited to be responsible for such a group, by introducing newcomers to regular attenders, offering refreshments and organising guest speakers if there is a topic the parents particularly want information about.

Semi-structured parenting courses can be run by health professionals for parents with preschool children. Such courses might be held at a GP surgery, a local community centre, in a room attached to a playgroup, nursery or infant school so that parents can attend the course while their children are elsewhere occupied on the same premises. The course agenda must reflect the needs of parents in the local community. Relevance is all – parents will come and recommend the course to other parents if the content is seen to be tailored to their particular concerns.

Different educational encounters provide the chance for different kinds of learning and none should be despised as too humble or embraced as the ultimate solution to providing learning opportunities for parents. Parenting courses assist with the development of problem-solving, decision-making and social skills. One-to-one encounters are opportunities to help increase parents' understanding of the situations in which they find themselves. Pamphlets and leaflets can provide useful information, as long as they are kept up to date.

When professionals are responsive to the needs of parents, they can play a significant part in building up parental resources. They are able to provide information and some of the support that used to come from the extended family in days gone by. The health professional as educator must, above all, be a reflective rather than an expert practitioner.

BOX 1.4	Differences between expert and reflective practitioners (based on Schon 1991:301)
Expert practitioner	Reflective practitioner
I am presumed to know, and must claim to do so, regardless of my own uncertainty.	I am presumed to know, but I know that I am not the only one in the situation to have relevant and important knowledge. I use my uncertainties as a source of learning for my clients and me.
I keep my distance from the client and hold on to my expert role. I give the client a sense of my expertise (conveying a feeling of warmth and sympathy as a 'sweetener').	I seek out connections to the client's thoughts and feelings. I allow her respect for my knowledge to emerge from her discovery of its relevance in her situation.
I look for status in the client's response to my professional persona.	I look for a sense of freedom and a feeling of real connection to the client as a consequence of no longer needing to maintain a professional façade.

Finally, the key to providing quality learning opportunities for parents is likely to be the sharing of successful ideas by educators. Too often in the past, good schemes have run in isolation from and in ignorance of each other, even when only a few miles apart. Reinventing the wheel is a waste of time and resources. As parenting programmes become increasingly accepted and demanded in our society, the need to evaluate (see Chapter 13) and to share good practice becomes paramount. Not to do so is to short change the parents whom we are seeking to serve.

KEY POINTS

- Parenting in the 21st century may be difficult because of the restrictions placed upon parents by adverse social circumstances and the disintegration of the extended family and local community.

- The world in which today's children are growing up is light years away from the world in which their parents grew up.

- Infants need empathic parents who tune in to the signals they are sending, intuit their needs and respond accordingly.

- The relationships between the mother and child, between the father and child and between the mother and father are equal in their influence on the child's development of trust, autonomy and initiative.

- Parents nurture the physical, emotional and spiritual well-being of their children by means of effective discipline, sensitivity to their psychological state, solving problems as they arise and providing positive reinforcement of desirable behaviour.

- Many parents are aware of the need to break the mould of parenting set in their own childhood.

- Health professionals can model good-enough parenting in their interactions with the families in their care, as well as encouraging and reassuring parents and so building their self-esteem.

REFERENCES

Ainsworth MDS 1989 Attachments beyond infancy. American Psychologist 44:709–716

Barlow J, Stewart-Brown S 2000 Understanding parenting programmes: the benefits for parents of a home-school linked parenting programme. Paper given at CPHVA Conference, July, London

Bee HL, Barnard KE, Eyres SJ et al 1982 Prediction of IQ and language skills from perinatal status, child performance, family characteristics and mother–infant interaction. Child Development 53:1134–1156

Bornstein MH 1995 Parenting infants. In: Bornstein MH (ed) Handbook of parenting. Volume 1: Children and parenting. Lawrence Erlbaum Associates, New Jersey, pp 3–39

Brockington I 1996 Motherhood and mental health. Oxford University Press, Oxford

Clement S 1995 'Listening visits' in pregnancy: a strategy for preventing postnatal depression? Midwifery II (2):75–80

Collins WA, Harris ML, Susman A 1995 Parenting during middle childhood. In: Bornstein MH (ed) Handbook of parenting. Volume 1: Children and parenting. Lawrence Erlbaum Associates, New Jersey, pp 65–89

Fagot BI 1995 Parenting boys and girls. In: Bornstein MH (ed) Handbook of parenting. Volume 1: Children and parenting. Lawrence Erlbaum Associates, New Jersey, pp 163–183

Family Policy Studies Centre 2000 Family change: guide to the issues. Family Briefing Paper 12. Family Policy Studies Centre, London

Fleissig A 1993 Are women given enough information by staff during labour and delivery? Midwifery 9:70–75

Flint C 1986 Sensitive midwifery. Heinemann, London

Gowen JW 1979 Poverty related developmental delay: is parent education the answer? Paper presented at the Ira J Gordon Memorial Conference on Parent Education and Involvement, University of North Carolina

Grimshaw R, McGuire C 1998 Evaluating parenting programmes: a study of stakeholders' views. National Children's Enterprises Ltd, London

Hadley A 2000 Tough choices: young women talk about pregnancy. The Women's Press, London

Henry M 1996 Young children, parents and professionals: enhancing the links in early childhood. Routledge, London

Illingworth PS 1991 The normal child, 10th edn. Churchill Livingstone, Edinburgh

Kennell J, Klaus M, McGrath S, Robertson S, Hindley C 1991 Continuous emotional support during labour in a US hospital. Journal of the American Medical Association 265:2197–2201

Maccoby EE 1984 Middle childhood in the context of the family. In: Collins WA (ed) Development during middle childhood: the years from six to twelve. National Academy of Sciences Press, Washington DC, pp 184–239

McIntosh J 1993 The experience of motherhood and the development of depression in the postnatal period. Journal of Clinical Nursing 2:243–249

Mortley E 1998 'Good enough' parenting: the role of parenting education. Social Work Monographs, Norwich

Nolan M 1997 Antenatal education: where next? Journal of Advanced Nursing 25:1198–1204

Oakley A 1980 Women confined. Martin Robertson, Oxford

Oakley A, Hickey D, Rajan L 1996 Social support in pregnancy: does it have long-term effects? Journal of Reproductive and Infant Psychology 14:7–22

Parke BD, Cassidy J, Burks VM, Carson JL, Boyum L 1992 Familial contributions to peer competence among young children: the role of interactive and affective processes. In: Parke RD, Ladd GW (eds) Family–peer relationships: modes of linkage. Lawrence Erlbaum Associates, New Jersey, pp 107–134

Parratt J 1994 The experience of childbirth for the survivors of incest. Midwifery 10:26–39

Pugh G, De'Ath E 1984 The needs of parents: practice and policy in parent education. Macmillan Education, Basingstoke

Rutter M 1981 Maternal deprivation reassessed. Penguin Books, Harmondsworth

Schon DA (ed) 1991 The reflective turn. Teachers' College Press, New York

Shapiro MC, Najman JM, Chang A, Keeping JD, Morrison J, Western JS 1983 Information, control and the exercise of power in the obstetrical encounter. Social Science and Medicine 17(3):139–146

Sosa MD, Kennell J, Klaus M, Robertson S, Urrutia J 1980 The effect of a supportive companion on perinatal problems, length of labor, and mother–infant interaction. New England Journal of Medicine 303 (11):597–600

Winnicott DW 1957 The child and the family: first relationships. Tavistock, London

RESOURCES

Home-Start UK
2 Salisbury Road, Leicester LE1 7QR
Tel: 0116 233 9955
Website: www.home-start.org.uk
Home-Start visitors are volunteers who work alongside the statutory health and social services, offering friendship, practical advice and support to families with young children who have come under stress.

National Childbirth Trust (NCT)
Alexandra House, Oldham Terrace, Acton, London W3 6NH
Tel: 020 8992 8637
Website: www.nctpregnancyandbabycare.com
The National Childbirth Trust offers information and support in pregnancy, childbirth and early parenthood. It aims to give every parent the chance to make informed choices.

NEWPIN
Sutherland House, 35 Sutherland Square, London SE17 3EE
Tel: 020 7358 5900
Works mainly in London and Northern Ireland, offering long-term support for families under stress, with the aim of breaking the cycle by which

destructive behaviour can be repeated in succeeding generations. It seeks to alleviate maternal depression and other mental distress while focusing on child–parent relationships and prevention of emotional abuse.

Parent Network
Parentline Plus, Third Floor, Chapel House, 18 Hatton Place, London
EC1N 8RU
Tel: 020 7284 5500
Website: www.parentlineplus.org.uk
Parent Network seeks to improve the quality of family life by enabling parents to improve relationships with their children. The core 30-hour course is structured so that parents can share experiences, remember what it is like to be a child, practise ways of listening to children and work out how to be clear and firm in making requests and setting boundaries. Parent Network has more than 200 facilitators working in 30 areas across the country. The facilitators are parents who have been trained in the course content and facilitation skills.

2 | Supporting adult learning

Elaine Spink

INTRODUCTION

We all have the ability, at any age, to change our lives through learning.
(Campaign for Learning 2000)

'Changing lives' is an enormous challenge for both the learner and the educator. As an educator you have the responsibility for ensuring that the changes are positive and purposeful. This requires a broad range of skills and understandings but the range is within the reach of most of us and can take us into the rewarding, dynamic and stimulating realm of adult learning.

To support and promote adults' learning effectively educators need to have considered the nature of learning itself, examined the skills involved in teaching adults, turned the spotlight upon themselves and their own learning and teaching styles and to have at their disposal a range of teaching strategies.

This chapter considers each of these aspects and offers support to you, the adult educator, in putting the principles into practice.

ADULTS LEARNING

The challenge is for you . . . to encourage all these people to acquire new skills and knowledge. You are more likely to do this well if you have an understanding of how people learn. (Priest & Schott 1991:11)

What is learning like?

Whether you are four or 94, the brain has an amazing capacity to learn. How this happens has been debated over centuries but what seems clear is that to be effective, learning has to involve learners. This may seem obvious but consider your own experiences of learning within educational settings. To what extent did you develop *understanding* of the things you learnt about, rather than simply knowledge of them? To what extent were your ideas and experiences, values and attitudes acknowledged? Many will have experienced the jugs-and-mugs approach to education (Brem 1996): the teacher is the jug, full of knowledge, and the students are the mugs to be filled. And yet time and time again, research and experience show that the more active the learners are, the more effective is the learning process; the more passive they are, the less deep will be the learning (Rogers 1996). Figure 2.1 illustrates this view.

FIGURE 2.1   *What do you learn?*

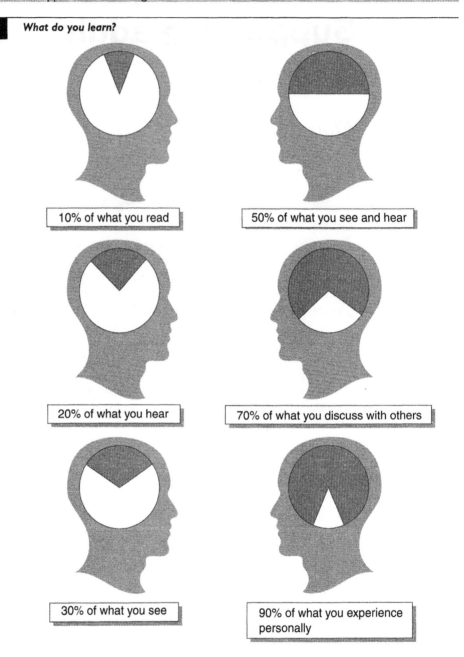

10% of what you read

50% of what you see and hear

20% of what you hear

70% of what you discuss with others

30% of what you see

90% of what you experience personally

There are many variations on this theme. They include the supposed ancient Chinese proverb 'I hear and I forget; I see and I remember; I do and I understand', to which we will return later, and an adage about learning skills (first told to me when working with educators in Indonesia but commonly known in other cultures too): 'Give a man a fish and you feed him for a day; teach a man to fish and you feed him for a lifetime'. Such phrases contain powerful messages for educators. They also demonstrate that there is little new ground to be broken here – the whys and wherefores of learning have exercised minds for thousands of years.

What is 'active learning'?

Active learning does not rely on 'action' in the sense of lots of physical activity (although this could feature in the learning) but rather on providing opportunities for learners to consider their own views, feelings and attitudes, to acknowledge personal experience, to use learning as the means of making sense of each person's world.

An influential view of learning (constructivism) holds that all individuals come to a learning situation with firmly held ideas, based on the experiences they have had so far. Learning happens when they question these ideas, look for alternatives, are exposed to ideas which better fit reality. The approach puts learners at the centre of the learning process with the teacher becoming a facilitator, not a giver of information. Learning certainly does not happen in a smooth, straight line, ever onward and upward. If you think of your own learning, you will be able to recall times when you did not seem to be learning very much at all, times when learning happened at a great pace and times when it even seemed to go backwards! (For example, I'm more confused now than when I started.) Your learning line is certainly likely to be wavy but chances are, if the constructivists are right, that it may also be U-shaped (Fig. 2.2).

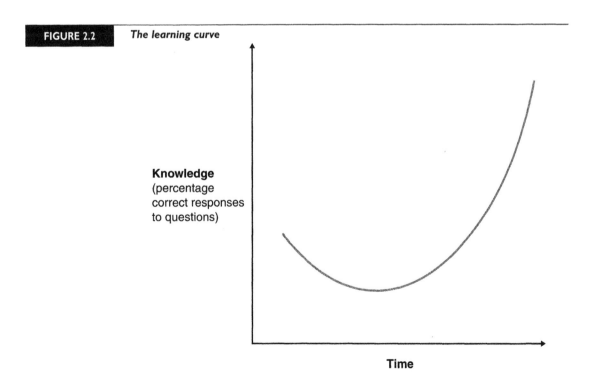

FIGURE 2.2   *The learning curve*

Knowledge
(percentage
correct responses
to questions)

Time

We arrive at a learning situation with some ideas about the topic area (almost never are we 'blank slates'). What happens next, with the activities/exercises/input the situation offers, is that we start to re-examine these ideas, to question what we thought we already knew, to wonder about our beliefs. All this doubting takes us into the 'trough of uncertainty' (i.e. the 'more confused than when I started' stage) and we *have* to go through this for learning to proceed and lead to new understandings. It's a healthy hole to be in! Unfortunately, this is where much education, for adults and children, stops. Time is up and we move on to a new topic or a new issue, leaving learners confused and appearing to understand less than when they arrived.

A good educator helps those she works with to climb out of the trough and to continue on the upward path. More about how she does this to follow . . .

In working with parents, you not only want to provide knowledge but also to encourage parents to develop deeper understanding, to enable them to develop skills or change attitudes. This demands a different approach from 'mug filling'.

Factors affecting learning

There is an enormous range of factors which can help or hinder us in learning. The following have all been found to be significant.

- The underlying philosophy of the educator. How do *you* believe people learn? This will influence all your interactions with learners.
- The environment. This includes both the setting (location, rooms, physical comfort) and the 'atmosphere' (levels of communication, degree of formality) (see p. 37).
- Methods of teaching and learning (discussed on pp. 42–46).

Learning styles

We have all been engaged in learning for the whole of our lives and will have developed our own preferred learning styles. The consensus from research is that there are (at least) four styles, as described in Box 2.1.

Andrea Robertson (1994) uses another common classification of learning styles – visual learners, auditory learners and kinaesthetic learners – and gives a useful breakdown of their characteristics and the implications for the educator.

Visual learners relate most easily to pictures, demonstrations, models, videos and written material. They use their imagination to create mental pictures. The educator needs to include lots of visual aids. Writing activities will also have appeal. Visual learners will need thinking time, to construct their mental images of the points you are making.

Auditory learners use their sense of hearing as their primary means of absorbing information. They enjoy verbal involvement, discussion and listening to others' experiences. They may look down or close their eyes when listening intently as they are not so reliant on eye contact. The educator should organise discussions and make use of tapes and/or videos.

Kinaesthetic learners learn from activities which engage all their senses and involve their whole body. They like practical sessions and physical movement.

BOX 2.1	*Learning style (based on Kolb 1984)*

Active learner
I act first and think later; I like lots of new experiences; I'll try to find out how things work before reading the instructions; I like to find out things for myself; I'm enthusiastic, I like meeting new people and experiencing new things.

Reflective learner
I am cautious and prefer to 'wait and see'. I look at things from different angles. I listen and take time to make up my mind. I like to know what others think before adding my own ideas.

Theorising learner
I like things to be logical. I enjoy analysing and looking for patterns, principles and models. Rules are good. I try to be objective and work things through step by step. I am not as comfortable with other people's feelings or different opinions.

Experimental learner
I am keen to try out new ideas and to put into practice things I have been told to see if they work. I like solving problems and meeting new challenges. I am energetic, confident and impatient if there is too much talk, not enough action.

Which one best describes you?

They generally respond well to touch. The educator should ensure there are practical aspects to each session and provide opportunities for handling resources.

Would that it were as simple as this . . . Of course, we rarely fall into one category exclusively and may indeed move from one to another, depending on the type of experience being offered.

The key word for educators is *variety*; we will come into contact with a huge variety of people and it is essential that this variety is reflected in our approaches and methods. The preferred learning styles of *everyone* should feature.

Barriers to learning

A recurring theme in this chapter will be the need to respond to those you work with as individuals, recognising their needs and abilities and building on these. This necessitates acknowledging the myriad factors which can affect learning, both positively, supporting and enhancing our abilities to develop new knowledge and skills, and negatively, impeding our progress. These 'barriers to learning' are common to all learners, although the causes may differ. The activities below encourage you to think of barriers to learning you have experienced and

ACTIVITY 2.1

Think of a situation when your learning did not progress as well as it might have (during a work-related course, at school, at college, at night classes, in leisure time). Can you identify reasons for the problems you experienced? Who or what made it difficult for you to learn?

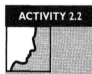

THE NIGHT CLASS

Ravi wanted to learn to play the classical guitar and enrolled for an evening course of 10 sessions at a high school. His daughter wished to use the car on the same evening so Ravi offered to travel to his classes by public transport. This meant two buses or a bus ride and a long walk. He arrived late for the first class (compounded by difficulties in finding the right room in the building) and noticed that he was by far the oldest member of the group. There were also many more people than he was expecting. The teacher said 'hello' and carried on with her talk. A class member smiled at Ravi and indicated the empty seat next to him, before leaning over and whispering 'Have you brought your sitar too?' Ravi felt exasperated.

The second class was better, although the tasks set by the teacher were very repetitive and the same for everybody.

Ravi decided to miss Class 3 – he was very tired after a particularly hectic day at work – and also missed Class 4 as he was needed at home that evening to take care of the younger children. In Class 5, Ravi struggled to catch up on the chords and practise pieces he had missed. The group was considerably smaller now but the teacher devoted most time to two 'star pupils'. Class 6 was better but Ravi realised his progress was slow. It was such an effort even to get there. He dropped out of the course that week.

What were the barriers to learning for Ravi?

then to analyse the barriers facing another individual. (The 'Ravi goes to night school' tale is based on a true story, although names have been changed.)

The barriers to learning for Ravi can be grouped into three categories (Maxted 1999):

- cultural
- social
- personal.

Cultural barriers include those relating to age, ethnic origin, gender and class (at least two of which were experienced by Ravi). Unemployment also falls into this category as a significant barrier to learning, carrying a cultural stigma. The education system itself is a barrier to learning in some cases, rooted as it is in information transfer rather than finding out.

Social barriers in the example described include the location and travel difficulties; the inadequate guidance and support given (from the lack of directions to guide people to the right room to the approach and attitude of the teacher); and childcare issues.

Personal barriers for Ravi were low motivation (not a normal feature of his personality but a reaction to the circumstances), lack of confidence, his perception of an age effect, tiredness and family pressures. The teaching and learning style was not suited to him. The result was a perceived lack of any reward (it's just not worth the effort) and a halt to learning.

The factors highlighted are some of the most common barriers to learning faced by adults and will undoubtedly impinge upon the parents you work with.

It is part of the role of the educator to assist learners to cross the barriers, jump the hurdles and find ways around the obstacles.

We (adult learners) can all be motivated to see learning as important if we can find the right kind of learning in a location and time which suits us (Maxted 1999). The 'right kind of learning' arises from a series of experiences, or interactions, and the 'right kind of teaching' is essentially about managing these interactions.

Learning occurs when a learner interacts in a *variety* of ways (because of the variety in learning styles) with other learners, with the content and with the educator (Fig. 2.3). The quality of these interactions determines the quality of the learning – and this relies on the skills of the educator. In moving on to consider principles in teaching adults, we begin to unravel what it means to be a 'good teacher'.

TEACHING ADULTS

What is different about teaching adults compared to teaching children? Adults undoubtedly have had longer to develop their attitudes (so perhaps they are more firmly entrenched), they have certainly had more experiences which could have formed barriers to learning and they will have clearly defined expectations about their educators and any courses they attend. Nevertheless, from everything previously discussed about the nature of learning, the answer to the initial question would appear to be 'very little'. The need for active involvement, the importance of each individual's ideas, the need to acknowledge variety in learning styles and attitudes to learning are highly significant whatever the age of the learner.

| FIGURE 2.3 | *Learning interaction* |

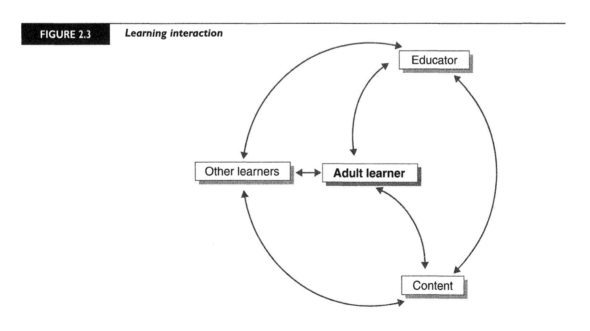

Teaching is a complex task. And yet it is a task we all know something about, from our own experiences as learners.

What makes a teacher effective? The following activity begins to pick out the features of effective teaching.

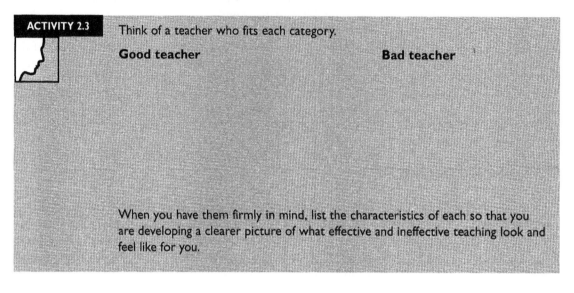

ACTIVITY 2.3

Think of a teacher who fits each category.

Good teacher   **Bad teacher**

When you have them firmly in mind, list the characteristics of each so that you are developing a clearer picture of what effective and ineffective teaching look and feel like for you.

Just as learning is essentially the same process for all learners, so teaching is essentially about developing and applying generic skills, whatever the ages of the learners. This makes it as relevant for you to examine the qualities of a teacher you particularly liked when you were five as to try to identify the skills of a teacher of adults.

When I first carried out this activity, it was surprising how quickly one individual came to mind as 'the best'. From informal research, it appears that most of us have one such teacher who stands out because of their particular combination of skills and attributes. There is much that can be learned from identifying their features.

Here are some of the characteristics of Mrs C.

BOX 2.2   *The good teacher*

- Treated class with respect
- Asked for our opinions
- Ran extra sessions
- Gave impression of knowing us well
- 'Really knew her stuff'
- Lessons were interesting
- Motivated everyone to do as well as possible
- Made difficult ideas easier to follow

These were the overt features of Mrs C's teaching, noted by all the pupils she worked with. But they were merely the lilies on the surface of a very deep pool! The apparent ease with which she 'made learning happen' belied the extent of her learned skills in the practicalities of teaching and of her natural skills in relating to people.

Her lessons were interesting as a result of careful planning and preparation and it was clear that she had specific learning outcomes in mind as she would inform us of what she hoped we would achieve during a lesson. Your interactions with adult learners should be planned and you need to look closely at your teaching. This can effectively be achieved by asking yourself three questions.

- What is the purpose of this piece of teaching?
- Why do I want to do it? (This will relate to your overall aims.)
- How can I best help the learners to achieve the purpose?

When you are clear about the 'what' and 'why' and have focused on providing variety in the 'how', almost inevitably your lessons are interesting.

Subject knowledge can be of great help in this respect too. This sounds obvious but is a point worth making as educators are sometimes required to teach in areas other than their own. Depth of subject knowledge gives you confidence in your teaching – and I am sure that it is this which learners respond to so positively ('really knew her stuff'). The content of what you teach needs to be meaningful for you too, if you are to make it convincing.

With hindsight, it is possible to see that Mrs C was slipping with apparent ease between a number of different roles. This is often the case with 'good' teachers. She was certainly a skilled planner and an efficient organiser, at times she was an instructor (imparting information) or a leader (encouraging, motivating, making decisions) or a counsellor (ready to listen and to support). At other times she was a group member, joining in with activities and finding things which were new to her too. Of necessity, she was also an assessor and evaluator, having the responsibility, as all educators do, of monitoring learners' progress and knowing how well things were going.

The ability to adopt different roles, usually in response to the needs of the learners, lies at the heart of effective teaching. Which hats will you be most comfortable wearing? And which will you need to take out of storage and dust off? You discover which hat to wear largely by watching and listening to the adults with whom you are working.

Our 'good teachers' were all, almost certainly, good communicators. Chances are that, like Mrs C, they listened as much as they talked and so learnt a great deal about those they worked with. They were skilled in 'reading the signs', understanding that much of the information we gain about other people comes from non-verbal cues (such as their posture and expressions), and so were able to give the impression of 'knowing us well'. This impression is strengthened by the quality of the feedback we receive from educators. Learners need positive feedback (for example, 'You made a really good point', 'That was great') but they also need *honest* feedback which includes guidance on the next steps to take. We can find it difficult to offer criticism, however constructive this is, but we are not helping learners by shying away from honest appraisal.

It may help to structure feedback into a sandwich – the 'appraisal sandwich' (Fig. 2.4) – where you begin with a positive comment (the top slice of bread), then make suggestions for improvements or identify the next steps (the filling) and finish with another positive comment (the bottom slice of bread).

The memorable teachers are usually those who motivated us and this is another key factor in their success.

FIGURE 2.4	*The appraisal sandwich*

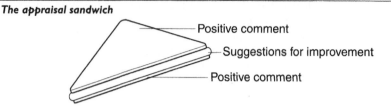

Without motivation, there can be no real learning. (Maxted 1999:6)

Unfortunately, this frequently seems to be overlooked, particularly in adult education. The National Adult Learning Survey (DfEE 1998) found that the most commonly cited obstacle to learning was lack of interest and motivation. These feelings translate into negative attitudes to learning, which are then transferred to people around us. It is therefore a matter of urgency for educators of parents to address issues of interest and motivation – a parent's attitude today may be a child's tomorrow.

Not all barriers to learning are easily overcome but Maxted (1999) recommends that we look *first* to motivation – 'the most necessary first step on the proverbial thousand mile journey' (p. 69).

If we create an appetite for learning everything else should gradually follow. Box 2.3 lists some of the requirements for adult learners if they are to be motivated by our teaching. It also outlines their expectations of the educator.

BOX 2.3	*Motivation*

To become or to stay motivated adults need to:
- know that they are respected as individuals in their own right
- feel secure and able to try things out
- see that their needs are being met, in relevant and appropriate ways
- know what they have to do
- be actively involved
- have feedback on how well they are doing
- feel they are getting 'a good return' on their investment (of time, money, effort).

Adults expect the educator to:
- be knowledgeable
- be a competent teacher
- practise what they preach (for example, listening, acknowledging individual differences, showing enthusiasm)
- recognise their status as adults and therefore treat them with respect and dignity.

Do all of these ingredients (the ability to plan, to evaluate, to appraise, to listen, to motivate, to build confidence and so on) add up to 'the good teacher'? Not necessarily.

There is something extra which binds the parts and, though hard to define, may best be described as professional empathy – the ability to respond to learners at their level and to understand their particular needs. This is shared by effective educators whether working with 3 year olds or 33 year olds.

Teaching adults is rarely easy. It has been said that in adult education there are no bad students; that if the adults fail to learn or if attendance falls off, this is because the teacher has not prepared an adequate programme or adopted appropriate teaching and learning methods (Rogers 1996). This may not always apply but the onus is certainly on the educator to try to ensure effective learning.

What sort of teacher – or educator – of adults will you be? The focus now turns very firmly to *you* . . .

UNDERSTANDING YOU

You are central to this consideration of adult learning and adult teaching. Everything that makes you 'you' will affect your role as an educator. Recognising your strengths and weaknesses will enable you to build upon those strengths and tackle those weaknesses. The better you know yourself, the more confident you will be and the more resources you will have to draw upon. *Appearing* confident is so important for educators. The genuine confidence which will come with teaching to your strengths and having the skills to respond to learners in a variety of ways will be an added bonus.

To understand yourself as an educator, you need to take a close look at your values and beliefs, your preferred learning styles and your own teaching style. Once you have done this, you will have practised many of the self-evaluation skills of importance to educators.

Your values and beliefs

As educators we most likely would all wish to feel we were objective, unbiased, unprejudiced. But very often, our values, beliefs, expectations and cultural norms are affecting our words and actions, often in quite subtle or subconscious ways. Have a look at the drawing in Activity 2.4 and complete the task.

With the best of intentions, it is very difficult (if not impossible) to respond to people neutrally. Personal viewpoints are highly influential.

You will be supporting adults in learning more about parenting and parenting is something *everyone* has experience of, whether as a parent themselves or having been parented. Your views will largely be based on your personal experiences and so will everyone else's, but their experiences will have been different. This gives rise to enormous potential for clashes of opinion. Parenting issues are emotionally charged and value laden.

It may be very valuable for you to debrief your own parenting experiences, with a friend or a counsellor. Once you are aware of your own feelings and have taken steps to resolve any particular issues, you will be in a much better position to support others objectively.

ACTIVITY 2.4

Jot down, as quickly and as fully as you can, your initial responses to this picture. (based on Drummond 1993)

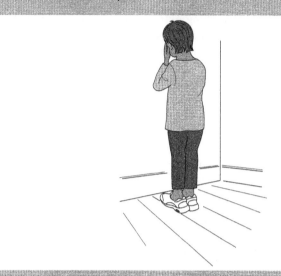

Now try to categorise your responses.

■ How many were *factual*, e.g. a corner, a person covering face?
■ How many were *interpretations*, e.g. 'a girl', 'a black person', 'crying', 'a child sent to stand in the corner'?
■ How many were *judgements*, e.g. 'a naughty child sent to the corner', 'a lonely girl, crying, with no-one to play with'?
■ What other interpretations could you make?
■ Is this child crying or being the 'seeker' in a game of hide and seek?
■ Can we be sure of the gender, race, location or feelings of this person? No, we can't and yet most of us read things into this picture for which there is no firm evidence.
■ What do you think made you make those interpretations?

> Sorting out your own joys and sorrows about birth and parenting will not only help you personally but will make unbiased comment, non-judgemental responses and open-minded approaches to problem-solving easier for you to model. (Robertson 1994:53)

The word 'model' used by Robertson is highly significant. In supporting adult learners, we should all be modelling – modelling good attitudes to learning, to problem solving, to working collaboratively. But how much more important is it for us as educators of *parents* to model parenting skills.

What skills do you think a parent should have? (see Activity 2.5 on p. 33).

If you believe that parents need to be good listeners; able to give fully of their attention; able to play; able to have conversations based on open, person-centred questions; able to show affection . . . then I suggest we should be modelling all the skills from your shopping list in our interactions with parents. (And that includes 'playing'! We have all 'played' with a new idea or a new gadget or played games. Adults need to play too.)

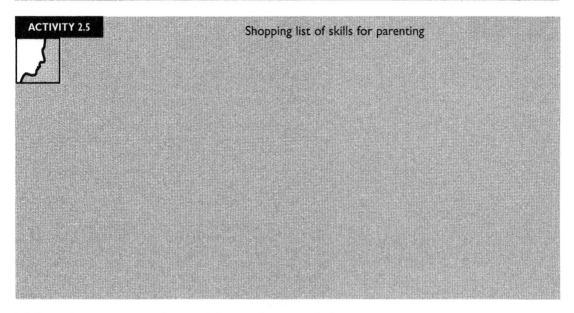

ACTIVITY 2.5   Shopping list of skills for parenting

What is your preferred learning style?

It is important to acknowledge your preferred style as your natural tendency will be to present material as you would like to receive it yourself in a learning situation (Robertson 1994). Alan Rogers (1996) goes further and says that as soon as educators feel unsure of themselves, threatened by inexperience, new material, lack of time or self-doubt, they automatically revert to the teaching methods by which they were taught. This is not always in the best interests of the learners and is something we must all watch out for.

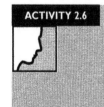

ACTIVITY 2.6   Think of a new skill or a new piece of knowledge you have learned in recent years.

■ Why did you learn this? (What was your motivation?)
■ What helped you to learn? (Which methods and approaches did you find helpful?)
■ What resources did you use?
■ How long did it take and what kept you going?

Read the descriptions of learners earlier in this chapter. Which do you think best describes you?

What kind of effect do you think your own preferred learning style will have on those you work with? More to the point, given the warning from Rogers (1996), what are you going to turn into when under stress and the clock strikes 12?

Your teaching style

Many attempts have been made to categorise the different styles educators adopt. Reading the four descriptions in Figure 2.5, which one do you feel is most likely to describe you?

| FIGURE 2.5 | *Teaching styles* |

The lion-tamer

Look, listen, behave yourself

You like to work from lists of objectives and a predetermined structure. This can seem rigid and narrowly focused but provides the familiarity and security some learners need. You often demonstrate and can explain things clearly from your perspective. You feel comfortable in a position of authority within a group and tend to be the centre of attention. Questions will be avoided if you feel you cannot answer them.

The doubter

What am I doing here?

You are still wondering how you got there and may be new to your role. You feel rather insecure in your knowledge, particularly of systems and procedures, and so will often refer questions on to 'a higher authority'. You tend to structure things a little loosely as someone may have a better method or idea than yours. You are uncomfortable with silence and so try to fill up the gaps.

The democrat

What do you want to do?

You recognise that there is variety in learners' experiences, beliefs and backgrounds and believe that they can therefore find their own paths. You encourage participation and learning from one another. You have sound subject knowledge and can put this across in a variety of ways, although you prefer learners to discover things for themselves. You readily admit to gaps in your knowledge and will leave agendas open to negotiation.

The expert

Let me show you the way

You know and understand a great deal about your subject. It can be difficult for you to relate to those who struggle to grasp concepts in your subject area. It can also be difficult for you to accept the views or ideas of others because you believe you are right, based on years of experience. You are keen for others to recognise the worth in what you are saying and doing. It is hard for you to accept criticism.

It can help to recognise general trends in our approaches to teaching, while acknowledging that we rarely sit in one box exclusively. If 'boxes' do not provide an adequate model of teaching styles, do other models have more to offer? It is common to see teaching styles represented as a continuum (Fig. 2.6).

There are some strengths to this view, recognising as it does that there are no hard and fast divisions between styles and that teachers can move along the continuum, in each direction, between the two extremes.

FIGURE 2.6

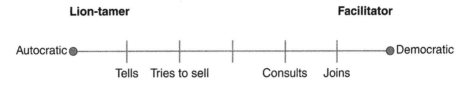

Continum of teaching styles (based on Rogers 1996)

However, there are problems with this model too as the implication is that the left side is 'bad' and the right side 'good'. And what are you if you are in the middle? It is wrong to assume that lion-tamers are poor teachers and facilitators the best teachers. The facilitator's style may not suit all learners: some may be uncomfortable with the degree of autonomy or with the idea of learning from other people or they may perceive a lack of structure. Perhaps these learners are happiest when told what to do or what to think – they need a lion-tamer!

There would seem to be two continua operating, giving rise to a third model (Fig. 2.7).

This gives many more possibilities and seems to better reflect the variety and disparity in teaching styles. You could be a doubting democrat, an expert autocrat, an expert democrat or a doubting autocrat – or rest on any point between. In the centre of this model would be the effective facilitator (or 'best teacher'), a person who is not 'sitting on the fence' but who can position themselves in any quadrant according to the demands of the learners or the situation. This teacher may be autocratic about some aspects of their teaching (especially about processes that they *know* to be effective) and completely democratic about content. They dip into different styles whenever appropriate.

The skills required to vary your teaching according to the context do not develop overnight. The key is to be prepared to make changes in the way you

FIGURE 2.7

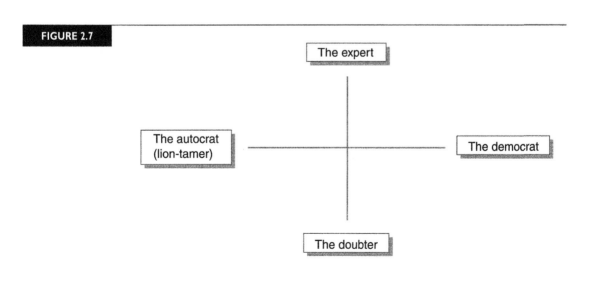

work with other people, to be aware that there are different styles which can be adopted and to know that there really is no excuse for *always* being a lion-tamer!

How are you doing?

Evaluation, including self-evaluation, is an important process for the educator to engage in. After every interaction between educator and learner(s), the educator needs to assess how well things went (see Fig. 2.8).

■ Were the learning outcomes achieved?
■ What were the positives and the negatives?
■ What changes need to be made?

This will ensure your practice sits firmly within the cycle of effective teaching.

You also need to look closely at yourself. This need not be time consuming – brief notes jotted on the plan or in your records will be fine, as long as you address how you *feel* (not just what happened) and possible next steps.

■ How did I feel?
■ What did I do well?
■ What reactions/responses did I notice?
■ What have I learned?

Who are you going to share these thoughts with? There will be times when you need to debrief before you can move on.

Look after yourself

The cliché 'look after number one' applies here and does not mean that educators should be selfish and out for their own gains! You need to develop your own support systems and ensure that your needs are being met, in order to avoid some of the stresses that go with wearing different hats and supporting others.

| FIGURE 2.8 | *Cycle of effective teaching* |

The educator plans, carries out the plan, assesses/reviews/evaluates, then re-plans

Plan

Review

Do

If you are to remain effective you, too, need time and attention. It's like looking after your bank account – if you don't make deposits there will be trouble. (Priest & Schott 1991:209)

You also need to model to parents that it is fine to ask for help, to look for ways to 'lessen the load' and to look after your own needs.

How will you keep your 'bank balance' healthy?

ORGANISING TEACHING AND LEARNING

As an educator of adults, you are responsible not only for *what* is taught but also for *how*. We have previously considered the effects of your philosophy (what you believe is effective learning and effective teaching) on those you work with. We now move on to consider the impact you can have on teaching and learning through your organisation of the following.

- Environment
- Grouping
- Timing
- Activities
- Resources.

If you are a fan of acronyms or mnemonics, this can, purely by chance, be recalled as GREAT!

Environment

Where will the teaching take place? (Remember the barriers to learning, one of the most common being difficulties with the location.)

- The location should be easily accessible and parking should be readily available. It should offer privacy and comfort. Are people likely to feel at ease there? (For example, not everyone feels comfortable, and therefore 'ready to learn', in hospital settings or places with an institutionalised feel.)
- Is it well lit and well ventilated?
- Are there access and facilities for disabled parents?
- Is there enough space for your purposes?
- How will you arrange the furniture? Everyone should be able to see everyone else (circles are best for this) and ideally should have similar chairs.
- Are toilet facilities adequate?
- Are refreshments available?
- Do you know where the emergency exits are? Ensure you pass this information on to the parent(s) you work with.

What will the 'atmosphere' be like?

- Aim to create a permissive atmosphere (Robertson 1994:57), where people feel free to talk and where they can be sure of respect and acceptance.

- Give a warm welcome, introducing yourself, ensuring any waiting time has been pleasantly spent (drinks, reading material).
- Learn names quickly (see 'Selecting strategies').
- Display enthusiasm for your role and for the subject matter.
- Give the impression of being quietly confident and enthusiastic (Daines et al 1993:109).

Grouping

Some of you will be supporting the learning of adults on a one-to-one basis, some will work with couples, others with small groups, yet others with large groups and for many, there will be a combination of all grouping formats. It is beyond the scope of this chapter to examine groups and group dynamics in great detail; the suggested reading will point you in the direction of further information and advice on dealing with particular issues and problems (such as 'the dominant group member' and 'non-participation'). However, general principles are offered here.

Working with individuals on a one-to-one basis brings its own challenges and pitfalls. It has the advantage that the individual receives your undivided attention and so her particular needs can be addressed. However, it is demanding for both because the educator *and* the 'learner' feel they have nowhere to hide, that all the attention is focused on how they are performing. Obviously, such an arrangement also means that the individual does not have the opportunity to learn from the experiences of others.

Small groups can provide richer opportunities for learning but a key question is 'When is a group not a group?' The answer is, when it is a number of individuals who just happen to be occupying the same space. This can frequently be observed in primary schools, where children are organised into groups but these 'groups' are simply individual children sitting around the same table. Group work implies collaboration and cooperation, working together towards a common goal. 'They [groups] help people reconsider and modify their attitudes and approaches, as well as producing more varied and more stimulating ideas than can individuals working alone' (Daines et al 1993:61). As we have already considered, attitude change may well be central to our work with adult learners, specifically parents, and so approaches which encourage this and also offer support and security (since change is often perceived as 'a risky business') *must* be a part of our repertoire. The development of groups begins with creating a sense of group identity. Tasks which help individuals to identify shared characteristics or experiences, enabling people to 'get to know one another', should be the forerunners to collaborative activities.

Four to six people is a comfortable size for a group since this provides a balance between pressure to join in and the opportunity to escape from the proceedings for a while. You can be temporarily overlooked but not totally forgotten!

Large groups can be time and resource efficient (the same content to many people at the same time) but require careful management if active learning is to operate successfully. Larger groupings offer too many hiding places – the learner can easily 'opt out'.

Timing

The timing of adult learning sessions can be crucial (and again, links with many of the barriers to learning already identified).

■ Does the timing exclude certain people from attending (e.g. those who work, those who pray at particular times)?
■ How can you minimise the impact on childcare arrangements?
■ Will the learners be 'fit to learn' (i.e. not too tired at the end of a long day or insufficiently awake at the start of a day)?

If you are planning sessions or classes, think carefully also about the timings of activities. Most adults have an attention span of about 5 minutes in any one burst. This makes maintaining attention quite a tall order for the educator, but one that is achievable with (and here comes that word again) *variety* in approaches and methods.

Activities/strategies/content

More detailed descriptions of activities and strategies follow under 'Your teaching session'. Three important principles underlying their organisation are:

■ they should build on existing knowledge and previous experiences
■ there should be variety (to accommodate different preferred learning styles)
■ they should make learning fun (thereby encouraging parents to model positive attitudes to learning with their children).

Resources

Using teaching resources, whether they be audio visual aids, materials, people, objects or events, not only makes the whole process more interesting and enjoyable but they actually do help teachers to teach more effectively and adult students to learn more efficiently. (Daines et al 1993:61)

Two key points for using resources are, first, that they are of good quality and second, that you are confident in using them. It helps to have a variety of resources to support each area of content (remember, they must appeal to visual, auditory and kinaesthetic learners).

If your work with adult learners takes you to different settings and locations, you may find it useful to put together a basic teaching kit. The contents of one such kit are listed in Box 2.4.

YOUR TEACHING SESSION

It may help to think of your teaching session in three sections and to plan carefully for each. This gives you the reassurance that you know what's coming next, while not needing to feel too constrained by a rigid plan.

BOX 2.4	*Educator's anything and everything kit*
A4 paper	Sellotape
Pens	Masking tape
Pair of scissors	Whiteboard pens
Pencils	String
Eraser	Tissues
Coloured marker pens	Notebook
Blank postcards	Flipchart paper
Highlighter pens	Glue stick
Blu-tack	OHP acetates
Paper clips	OHP pens
Sticky labels	Spare OHP bulb

1. How will you begin?
2. Which teaching strategies will you use?
3. How will you conclude?

The following general guidance points apply whether you are working with individuals or groups.

How to begin

The session – and particularly the first session – needs a good introduction.

> How you present and manage the first five minutes of a session will set the tone of what is to follow. (Daines et al 1993:114)

You may choose to introduce yourself, ensure the participants are aware of the 'comfort details' (toilets, refreshments and so on) and give an overview (briefly) of the session so that the participants know what is in store for them. (Anxiety is generated by fear of the unknown.) The focus will be entirely on you during this time but, as you are going to be modelling good 'people skills' and effective approaches to teaching and learning, it is much better to keep the passive audience parts to a minimum and encourage participation and action as soon as possible. This will lead you to . . .

The *warm-up* or *ice-melter* activity (sometimes referred to as an 'ice breaker' but melting best describes the process you will be trying to facilitate, rather than images of breaking or smashing down reserves!). Ideally, this activity should give everyone a chance to speak, it should be simple and it should be enjoyable. The rewards are that people begin to get to know one another and to identify common experiences; the individuals (including the educator) begin to form into a group and it sets the tone of what is to follow (less of you and more of them!).

Name rounds are commonly used to achieve the above and there are many variations on this theme. You could try:

- name plus something you like
- name plus favourite time of year
- name plus something good about the week.

If working with a group, you could invite them to form pairs (with a person they do not know) and to talk for a few minutes, finding out about the other person. Each individual then feeds back to the whole group the name of their 'partner' and something about them. When groups meet regularly over a period of weeks, the name round will become unnecessary after a couple of sessions. However, a warm-up activity (what Priest & Schott (1991) refer to as 'a settling exercise') can remain very beneficial for group relationships.

Figure 2.9 contains some suggestions for 'starters'.

The third element of 'How to begin' is negotiation. Participants and educator need to negotiate the ground rules, perhaps the content, find where the boundaries are, discover expectations and needs. Much of this can come to light through questioning and discussion (if working with individuals or pairs) or through a group activity (see below) if working with larger numbers.

Essentially, it is very valuable for you to know what the participants hope to *gain* from the session(s), what they could *give* to it, what would make a session *ghastly* for them and what *ground rules* they would like to see operating – the Four Gs (from Fletcher & Buggins 1997). An example of a chart produced from this agenda-setting activity is shown in Box 2.5.

The challenge for the educator is then to make sure that all the Four Gs are acknowledged and, wherever possible, acted upon.

Negotiation and agenda setting have to happen in the early stages of your work with a new group of people but not necessarily at the beginning of a session. It is hard to share hopes and concerns with people you barely know.

Practise what you will be preaching and encourage active involvement in teaching and learning activities first.

FIGURE 2.9

It's fun to ......

                             Being a mum means ......

    I would like to have been ......

                                  Nothing is so frustrating as ....

       As a child I ......

                        A good thing that happened to me this week was ......

Ten years from now ......

                            I really hate it when ......

      This week my child(ren) ......

| BOX 2.5 | *The Four Gs* |

Context: six couples in a 'Preparation for Parenting' course, working in two groups. All contributions were recorded on poster paper under the four headings.

Gains	*Gives*
Information	I'll listen
Good ideas	Support
Support	Friendship
Advice	Share experiences
	Give information

Ghastlies	*Ground rules*
(Or 'Gulp – oh no!)	
	Finish on time please
Being told what to do	Confidentiality
Do-gooders	Accept everyone's ideas
Role play	Don't judge
Airy-fairy ideas	

Selecting strategies

There are so many to choose from! (See Figure 2.10.) Rogers (1996:187) relates the tale of a group of teachers producing a list of 49 different teaching and learning strategies during a brainstorming activity and not exhausting all possibilities. How do you decide which ones to use? This will depend upon the number of people you are working with, their needs and preferred learning styles

| FIGURE 2.10 | *Teaching strategies* |

(found out by observing, by listening to what they say, by questioning and discussing) and your preferred style. Of course, the Chinese proverb outlined earlier (I hear and I forget, I see and I remember, I do and I understand) will influence your decisions. In the discussion of the strategies which follows, this has been translated into 'Tell me and I forget; show me and I remember; involve me and I understand', in order to place the emphasis on what the educator should do to support learning.

Figure 2.10 shows a range of teaching strategies, all of which could be used in your work with adults. A selection is considered in more detail but for comprephensive discussion you will need to refer to the texts in Further Reading and particularly to Daines et al (1993).

Discussion

> Discussion is a planned for and managed event where a group of people jointly explore a topic, area of knowledge or a set of attitudes. (Daines et al 1993:49)

It is a strategy with a lot to offer as meeting other people and sharing knowledge and experience are some of the most enjoyable features of adult education. Through discussion, people can express what they think or feel and acknowledge shared problems and beliefs (Priest & Schott 1991:71). But good discussions rarely just happen. They need preparation and what Priest & Schott aptly call choreography to keep them going. You need to find the trigger for a discussion, often an open question, based on feelings or opinions; for example, 'What do you think about . . . . ?' or 'How do you feel when . . . . ?'

Problems can arise. For example, what would you do about the silent person? Or the non-stop talker? Particular strategies for these cases include using a 'round' so that everyone has the opportunity to talk, breaking into smaller groups so that the quiet person may feel less intimidated and the talker has a smaller audience, positioning people carefully so that you can catch the eye of the quiet person and avoid catching the eye of the noisier one! A discussion should not be allowed to fizzle away. Bring it to a conclusion, once all who wish to contribute have done so, with a summing up and then a clean break, moving on to a different activity.

The lecture/talk: 'tell me and I forget'

This cannot be the whole story as there is still a place for lectures and talks in active learning. They can be effective ways of presenting information in a limited time and their familiarity to adult learners can put participants at their ease (as it is what they may be expecting). A useful method is simply to follow the structure for a session as outlined already (with an introduction, the key activities/points and a conclusion).

- *The 'lead-in'* – to capture interest and start people thinking about the subject. It may be a question, an anecdote, a picture or an object.
- *The key points* – clearly made and illustrated with appropriate resources and/or visual aids.
- *The summary* – recaps on the key points and 'ties up the ends'; for example, answering your initial question or returning to the open-ended anecdote.

It is worth bearing in mind that even the most attentive of people are unlikely to be listening fully beyond 20 minutes (and usually for less time than that). So set yourself time limits.

Some of the potential pitfalls in giving a talk, to however large or small an audience, include having to deal with drifting attention and resisting the temptation to read or recite from your script. The first can be overcome by introducing some participative activities, using a visual aid or you moving about more (within reason!). The second tends to arise from your own lack of confidence, so try to trust in your knowledge of the subject matter (you do not really need a script and your audience were not familiar with its content anyway and so will not know if you have left sections out). It can help to use prompt cards only (not your full notes) and to talk to visual aids (for example, pictures or overhead projector slides).

Remember that people respond to speakers who are warm, enthusiastic and stimulating. So smile and try to look as if you enjoy both the subject and the opportunity of sharing it with others. (Daines et al 1993:41)

Demonstration: 'show me and I remember'

Demonstrations are particularly useful in developing skills. Adult learners will benefit from watching you carry out a process and then having a go themselves or going along with you, copying your actions. Your skill may make the process look easier than it is (for example, changing a baby's nappy) so it helps to have thought stages through beforehand and broken them down into bite-sized chunks. Asking one of the participants to demonstrate can be effective too, but not if they feel they are being tested or 'judged'. Avoid this by asking the others to guide the demonstrator through the process. This then involves everyone. Demonstrations, even with high-quality resources and step-by-step explanations, should never be a substitute for practical activity, involving everyone in a 'hands-on' way.

Practical activity: 'involve me and I understand'

You can only be sure you have acquired a skill by practising it. And there is strong support for the view that you can only be sure you understand something if you can *apply* your knowledge in a variety of ways and situations (that is, be able to make the connections between separate pieces of knowledge and see the implications). Some of these situations, for skills and knowledge, must include practical activity. There are many advantages of practical work for adult learners. It encourages active participation and cooperation, enables people to learn from one another and provides opportunities for practising skills in a safe environment (it does not matter if things go wrong as the situation is not 'real').

I have kept the definition of 'practical activity' deliberately broad in order to encompass just about everything which is not sitting in a chair, listening to someone talk ('jugs and mugs'). Practical activity with your adult learners may involve sorting activities (e.g. words on cards to be sorted into groups), producing posters, making a model, drawing a cartoon, solving a problem by discussing case studies, role playing and scores of others. The decision is yours.

The following are the main forms of practical group activities from which you may wish to select. With the exception of role play, definitions and brief descriptions only are offered here; again, there is much in the literature on the details of each (see Further Reading).

Role play and simulation

Role play as a method of learning is often misunderstood. It may be perceived as acting or performing due to poorly structured or debriefed previous experiences. It may have led to people feeling uncomfortably self-conscious. Whatever the specific causes, role play is dismissed by some as a method of learning. And yet it is unhelpful to think of role play and simulation as 'just drama'. Their particular strength is that they offer: 'an opportunity for experiential learning in a safe context . . . with all the dynamics and characteristics of "real life" without any of the consequences' (TACADE 1983:7).

Role play can be very effective in practising skills and in exploring feelings (for example, 'How would you feel if your child said . . . ?'). It can be a powerful stimulus for attitude change, especially if taking on the roles of people with views different from your own. Research has shown that when asked to prepare a case in support of something to which they were opposed, adult learners were far more likely to modify their attitudes towards the issue (Shallcross 1995). Role play need not involve acting at all but trying to see something through the eyes of someone else. Give it a go!

Brainstorming

A group produces a comprehensive list of ideas and suggestions on a particular theme, with every contribution included.

Buzz group

Pairs or trios are asked to discuss, very briefly, a particular point or question.

Snowballing

An individual lists three or four points then joins with another person. This pair selects three points from their combined list and takes these to another pair. Two points are selected. Pairs become groups of four, then fours become groups of eight and so on until there is one list of three or four points for the whole group.

Games

Large or small groups use commercial or 'home-made' games, focusing on problem solving, decision making or team work.

Case studies and problem-solving exercises

A situation is described in written form for the group to analyse or solve the problems.

Work between sessions

Participants are asked to carry out a task between meetings, to give continuity and to maintain interest.

Strategies particularly useful for a one-to-one situation include discussion, case studies and/or problem-solving scenarios and guidance on individual practice. If working with larger groups (12 and above) the space available could push you towards a more static session. But knowing what you do about adult learning and appreciating that variety and participation are vital, this is less likely to have a negative impact on those you work with! It is possible to include participatory methods with large groups (Daines et al 1993:118) and for the learning to be more effective as a result. Strategies which can be adapted for large numbers include buzz groups, debates, brainstorms, case studies, discussions and small group practical tasks (which are not too demanding in terms of equipment or resources), with the groups formed from 4–6 people already sitting close to one another.

Some of the strategies discussed will inevitably hold more appeal over others for you and for those you work with. But, as has so often been the case in issues discussed here, variety is the key guiding principle if the strategies are to support learning; variety both in strategies *and* in the ways in which they are used. It would be useful to return to Figure 2.10 and think about who each strategy in the list is focused upon. Is it primarily a teacher activity, a group activity or an individual learner activity? Is there balance between the three in sessions you plan?

Concluding the session

Effective conclusions to teaching sessions are about helping people to recognise what they have achieved, motivating them to continue with their learning, gathering some feedback on what they thought of the session and looking forward to what will come next. This is a tall order unless you have allowed sufficient time for this to happen. Be warned that conclusions frequently 'drop off the end' of a session! There should also be 'time for talk', a part of the session, usually at the end, which gives opportunities for participants to speak to you on a one-to-one basis.

> How you end a session and talk with people afterwards can powerfully affect their motivation to achieve and to continue learning. (Daines et al 1993: 114)

In summary, the facts that there is no one right way to organise a teaching session and there is no one perfect teaching strategy which will 'do it all' mean that our search for effective organisation and strategies is unlikely to harm the learners. Our approaches and methods only become barriers to learning if they are limited in range and not adapted to needs.

WHY IS LEARNING SO IMPORTANT?

The government's response would focus on its economic worth: 'Education is the best economic policy we have' (Rt Hon Tony Blair MP). The Campaign for Learning (2000) emphasises the importance of moving with the times:

> In the 21st century, the new disadvantaged will be those who do not have the capacity to learn. They will sink, unable to change and adapt as they are flooded with ever more information and change.

But learning is essentially about individuals and the benefits it can bring to those individuals, their families and their communities. It can lead to personal growth and expanded horizons and enable people to create their own futures (Campaign for Learning 2000), all admirable aims for the educator to aspire to and all centred on increasing happiness.

> Learning brings more happiness than having sex, playing or watching sport or doing the National Lottery. (Gallup/North Yorkshire TEC 1997, quoted on Campaign for Learning website, 2000)

Spread a little happiness amongst the adult learners you work with!

KEY POINTS	
	■ Learning is an active, not a passive, process.
	■ Learners' previous experiences and ideas matter.
	■ Many factors, both internal and external, can affect learning and must be considered by the educator.
	■ There is variety in preferred learning styles.
	■ Teaching adults necessitates taking on many different roles.
	■ Your values and beliefs are highly influential.
	■ There is great variety in teaching styles and strategies – be guided in your selection by the needs of the adult learners.
	■ Learning should be an enjoyable experience for all those involved.

REFERENCES

Brem C 1996 Returning to learning? Studying as an adult: tips, traps and triumphs. Allen and Unwin, New South Wales, Australia

Campaign for Learning 2000 *http://www.campaign-for-learning.org.uk*

Daines J, Daines C, Graham B 1993 Adult learning, adult teaching. Continuing Education Press, Nottingham

Department for Education and Employment (DfEE) 1998 National Adult Learning Survey. DfEE, London

Drummond MJ 1993 Making assessment work: values and principles. Early Childhood Unit, Nottingham

Fletcher G, Buggins E 1997 The VOICES project: training and support for maternity services user representatives. Becoming an effective user representative. National Childbirth Trust, London

Kolb DA 1984 Experiential learning: experience as the source of learning and development. Prentice-Hall, London

Maxted P 1999 Understanding barriers to learning: a guide to research and current thinking. Campaign for Learning, London

Nolan M 1998 Antenatal education: a dynamic approach. Baillière Tindall, London

Priest J, Schott J 1991 Leading antenatal classes: a practical guide. Butterworth Heinemann, Oxford

Robertson A 1994 Empowering women. ACE Graphics, New South Wales, Australia

Rogers A 1996 Teaching adults, 2nd edn. Oxford University Press, Buckingham

Shallcross AG 1995 Accentuate the negative to latch onto the positive (how to save mockingbirds). Environmental Education Research 1 (3): 279–290

TACADE (Teachers' Advisory Council on Alcohol and Drug Education) 1983 Working with groups: supplementary materials. http://www.tacade.com/Tacade/Publications.html

FURTHER READING

Campaign for Learning: http://www.campaign-for-learning.org.uk

General learning principles, plus information on national events, contacts and further support.

Daines J, Daines C, Graham B 1993 Adult learning, adult teaching. Continuing Education Press, Nottingham

For detailed information, ideas and support for all aspects of planning and running adult learning sessions.

Nolan M 1998 Antenatal education: a dynamic approach. Baillière Tindall, London

Clear information on planning adult learning sessions, particularly the writing of aims and intended outcomes.

Robertson A 1994 Empowering women. ACE Graphics, New South Wales, Australia

3 Parenting education in schools

Olivia Montuschi

INTRODUCTION

This chapter begins by looking at the recent history of teaching about parenting in schools and examines the impetus and motivation behind the current government's enthusiasm for a new Personal, Social and Health Education (PSHE) curriculum to include parenting. It then moves on to examine some of the broader objectives and reasons for preparing children and young people for the parenting role. Drawing on recent key publications, and set out in question and answer form, the chapter concludes with guidance regarding the fundamental components of education for parenting, ways in which parenting education might be approached at different key stages, the appropriateness of the subject for boys and girls and children with special needs, and what schools and those preparing to teach parenting education need to have in place. There is an extensive, though not exhaustive, list of essential and recommended reading, resources for direct use in schools and useful contacts and addresses at the end.

BOX 3.1	*Key stages explained*

Key stages (defined precisely in section 355(1) a–d of the Education Act 1996) are the four stages of the National Curriculum as it applies to pupils of compulsory school age in all state, voluntary aided and voluntary controlled schools. The National Curriculum does not statutorily apply to independent schools. For each subject and for each key stage, programmes of study set out what pupils should be taught and attainment targets set out the expected standards of pupils' performance. It is for schools to choose how they organise their school curriculum to include the programmes of study.

■ Key Stage 1 applies to children between 5 and 7.
■ Key Stage 2 applies to children between 7 and 11.
■ Key Stage 3 applies to children between 11 and 14.
■ Key Stage 4 applies to children between 14 and 16.

PSHE is not a statutory subject but guidelines for programmes of study at the different key stages are included in *The National Curriculum: Handbook for Primary Teachers in England Key Stages 1 and 2* and *The National Curriculum: Handbook for Secondary Teachers in England Key Stages 3 and 4*.

BACKGROUND AND HISTORY

The idea of educating children and young people in school about their likely future role as parents is not a new one, as reported by Philip Hope and Penny Sharland in their report *Tomorrow's Parents* (1997). Sir Keith Joseph, who was Secretary of State for Social Services in the early 1970s, gave significant support to a major initiative on parenting and the DHSS followed this lead in promoting the idea of preparation for parenthood in schools. In 1977 the Select Committee on Violence observed that 'Much more should be done in the school curriculum to ensure that all pupils receive some education in the skills of parenthood' and another Select Committee recommended that 'the Government should ensure that education for parenthood is available for all boys and girls of all levels of intellectual ability' (quoted in Hope & Sharland 1997).

Various practical projects were set up by educational institutions and charities promoting the welfare of children and families but failed to thrive in the climate of the 1980s which deemed parenting to be a matter of private concern in which the state should not interfere. Education for parenting, instead of being available to all as had been envisaged, became a low-status option for less able children (mostly girls) where they learned *parentcraft* skills to do with caring for babies, rather than the broader role of preparing to be parents by reflecting on family relationships in their current lives.

In the early 1990s interest in parenthood education revived in response to growing concern about children's behaviour and the perceived 'failure' of parents to control their children. Once again, Keith Joseph, now ennobled, was at the forefront of public discussion and led a debate in the House of Lords. The questions he posed were:

> Would better preparation for parenthood offer some protection against a range of social ills in the future, such as antisocial behaviour of young men, teenage pregnancy, and family breakdown, and promote good behaviour in the classroom, educational attainment and the long-term health and welfare of children?

Under the spotlight trained on parenting in the 1990s, parents themselves began to emerge from their private struggles and admit that being a parent was probably the hardest task they had ever undertaken. The psychotherapist and author Susie Orbach said at a 1994 lunchtime seminar of the parent support charity Exploring Parenthood: 'The job of parenting is very hard and until recently it's been idealised – we've put a gloss on it. It's absolutely right that people are finally talking about how difficult parenting is'.

In the same year the Calouste Gulbenkian Foundation decided to fund a pilot project in five Manchester schools based on materials written by Philip Hope, then an independent consultant and now an MP. These materials were called Education for Parenthood and consisted of five booklets containing 28 classroom and community-based activities designed to encourage participative and experiential learning about parenthood. *Tomorrow's Parents* (Hope & Sharland 1997), the report of this highly successful pilot project, clearly had an impact on thinking about education in the Labour Party, then in opposition. Almost as soon as the Labour Party came to power a White Paper, *Excellence in Schools* (DfEE 1997), stated: 'We want all secondary schools to help teach young people the skills of good parenting, both formally and through contact with good adult role models' (para. 44).

In May 1998, the government announced that there would be a comprehensive review of the school curriculum to include PSHE. Citizenship and parenting were two subjects particularly singled out as being important to include. The broad aims of the new National Curriculum, the PSHE component of which started to be put in place in September 2000, are set out below.

- The school curriculum should aim to provide opportunities for all pupils to learn and to achieve.
- The school curriculum should aim to promote pupils' spiritual, moral, social and cultural development and prepare all pupils for the opportunities, responsibilities and experiences of life.

The two aims in fact reinforce each other. It has long been recognised that personal development facilitating the establishment of high self-esteem, the ability to see situations from the perspective of others and the capacity to reflect on one's own actions and behaviour and take responsibility for them play a significant part in the development of self-discipline, motivation and eventual achievement. Providing opportunities to learn and achieve essentially means supporting personal development.

The components of personal development mentioned above are also core qualities required in effective and responsible parenting. The development of these qualities forms a significant part of the content of the 'Developing good relationships and respecting differences between people' strand of the PSHE curriculum at Key Stages 1 and 2 (primary school) where the parenting element is implicit. At Key Stages 3 and 4 (secondary school) the knowledge, skills and understandings gained earlier can be built on with a more explicit focus on the functions of the family and roles of parents.

Two Steps Ahead: Fitting Parents for the Future (Parenting Education and Support Forum 1998) describes the differences between 'implicit' and 'explicit' parenthood education.

The *implicit* curriculum attends to the core or necessary skills which must be in place to enable people to fulfil their parenting role effectively. These skills are generic in that they are common to and transferable between the different strands of the PSHE curriculum. For example, work on building a sense of self and self-efficacy moves naturally to developing reflective, creative, social and decision-making skills. Not being exclusive to parenting, these skills do not require an overt 'parenting' identity and at Key Stages 1 and 2, that label need not be used.

The *explicit* curriculum at Key Stages 3 and 4 covers information, skills and situations particular to parenting. Young people will be invited to reflect on their future role as parents. The way of thinking about the role of parents will move from experiential, 'what is', to more cognitive, 'what will be' learning in parallel with other areas of the curriculum.

An example of implicit parenting input in the primary school curriculum is circle time which is used in many schools as a time to focus on recognising feelings, thinking about how other people feel and raising pupil self-esteem. In *PASSPORT: A Framework for Personal and Social Development* (Lees & Plant 2000), the report of a 2-year project commissioned by the Gulbenkian Foundation, there appears the following example from Christ Church School.

| BOX 3.2 | ***Primary school PSHE activity*** |

In this 20-minute weekly circle time session, 23 reception class pupils sat in a large circle with the teacher and classroom assistant. They participated in the following sequence of activities.

- Song: This is circle time.
- There's an empty chair next to me and I'd like . . . to sit next to me because . . . About five pupils took turns to choose someone to sit next to them.
- Round: I am wonderful!
- Closing with a song and a smile.

The following example of an 'explicitly' parenting-focused activity comes from *Parenting Perspectives: A Guide to Teaching Parenting Skills* (Howell et al 1997).

| BOX 3.3 | ***Secondary school PSHE activity – Parent wanted*** |

Pupils are invited to read the following advertisement with a partner.

Wanted: a responsible person, male or female, to undertake a lifelong project. Candidates should be totally committed, willing to work up to 24 hours a day, including weekends during the initial 5-year period. Occasional holidays possible but may be cancelled without notice. Knowledge of health care, nutrition, psychology, child development, household management and the education system essential. Necessary skills: communication and listening, negotiation and problem solving, stress management and conflict resolution, budgeting and time management, decision making, ability to set boundaries and priorities as well as providing loving support. Necessary personal qualities: energy, tolerance, patience, good self-esteem, self-confidence and a sense of humour. No training given or experience needed. No salary, but very rewarding work for the right person.

Discuss it in the class and ask pupils to complete an accompanying worksheet which asks them to identify in their own words five jobs that the applicant will have to do and then describe five skills they will need.

The activity can be supported with a range of advertisements – those for military personnel, the police and top secretaries make interesting starting points because of the skills and qualities required which may be contrasted with the skills and qualities required of an effective parent.

Follow-up and/or homework

EITHER   Design an advertisement for the job of parent that could appear in a newspaper magazine supplement, using desktop publishing software to make it look authentic.

OR   Write a science fiction story about a future where parents are suddenly in short supply after global pollution makes most of the population infertile. Imagine that you are one of the few people left who can breed the next generation.

There are three new national curriculum frameworks in the area of Personal, Social and Health Education and Citizenship.

- PSHE and Citizenship for Key Stages 1 and 2.
- PSHE for Key Stages 3 and 4.
- The statutory order for Citizenship for Key Stages 3 and 4.

The four strands which run through all the above frameworks are:

- Personal Development – developing children's and young people's confidence and responsibility and making the most of their abilities
- Active Citizens – preparing to play an active role as citizens
- Health and Safety – developing a healthy, safer lifestyle
- Relationships – developing good relationships and respecting the differences between people.

Although the government has made it clear that it believes parenthood education to be an important part of PSHE, it is only Citizenship and Sex and Relationships at Key Stages 3 and 4 which are statutory requirements and only Citizenship at these stages where there is a statutory programme of study. Schools are free to balance the remaining recommended strands of PSHE and develop the content of their chosen modules as they wish.

Components of the four strands above have been identified as:

- citizenship
- sex and relationships
- drugs
- sustainability (environmental education)
- work
- careers
- safety
- financial capability
- parenthood.

Non-governmental bodies have also had an important role in developing thinking around education for parenting. In September 1998, the Parenting Education and Support Forum issued a paper drawn up by its Parenthood Education in Schools working party, called *Two Steps Ahead: Fitting Parents for the Future*. This paper succinctly sets out the reasons why education for parenthood is so important in the context of the times we live in, what it needs to consist of, what it might hope to achieve and probably most important of all, who should teach it and the style in which it should be taught. In this, it builds on the experience of teachers in the pilot project in Manchester documented by Philip Hope and Penny Sharland in *Tomorrow's Parents* (1997). The influence of this short but significant pamphlet is clear in both the guidelines issued by the DfEE on Parenthood Education (forthcoming) and the final report of the PASSPORT project (Lees & Plant 2000).

PASSPORT: A Framework for Personal and Social Development, funded by the Calouste Gulbenkian Foundation, is a comprehensive guide to developing a whole-school approach to personal and social development within the framework of the new PSHE curriculum and in line with the recommendations of the National Healthy School Standard (DfEE 1999). Emphasis is placed on starting with the needs of pupils in each year group, the importance of equality and inclusion of all students and the value of allowing time for planning and reflection as part of the learning process.

The National Healthy School Standard aims to promote mental and physical health by adopting a whole-school approach that achieves a better match between a school's stated values and its provision. It is designed to complement and support the new PSHE framework. Each geographical area has a programme coordinator who is available to help individual schools tailor their own healthy school programme to meet local needs. There are three documents which are published by the DfEE as part of the Healthy School Standard:

- *National Healthy School Standard. Getting Started: A Guide for Schools*
- *National Healthy School Standard – A Practitioner's Guide*
- *The Healthy School Standard*: information on what being a healthy school is about for staff, parents, governors, pupils and community partners.

In 2001, the DfEE issued *Parenthood Education: Guidance for Schools*, designed to offer support and help to all those preparing to teach the different strands of the new PSHE curriculum. This excellent booklet, which sets out why it is important for schools to tackle the topic of parenthood, how to place it in the context of PSHE and Citizenship and how to deliver it successfully, is essential reading for anyone involved in devising a PSHE curriculum containing an element of parenting.

WHY PARENTING EDUCATION NOW?

The government's stated aim of promoting pupils' spiritual, moral, social and cultural development provides an obvious context for the current focus on teaching about parenting in schools. The interest, however, in this area of children's education and development does not come out of the air. Increasing concern about family breakdown, youth crime and the failure of the teenage pregnancy rate to drop alongside that of the USA and the rest of Europe has compelled the government to stray into an area once considered the private domain of individual families. Understandably, there is resentment and anxiety in some quarters that it is largely only family groupings which deviate from a narrow 'norm' which are the target of government interest. However, this should not be allowed to detract from what is truly ground breaking about the current focus on parenting: that for the first time there is acknowledgement at a high level that what goes on between parents and children makes a difference to the next generation's capacity to take their place as citizens and parents of the future.

Whilst the government's fundamental motivation may be apprehension about youth crime figures, the numbers of single parents on benefits and the costs of family breakdown, it is this recognition of the importance of the parenting relationship, particularly in the very early years, which has spawned important projects such as SureStart and the focus on education for parenting in schools.

The non-governmental bodies, whilst acknowledging the crucial importance of relationships between parents and children, have a more subtle and perhaps fundamental agenda. The PASSPORT project and the interest in education for parenthood of organisations such as the Children's Society, the Parenting Education and Support Forum and Antidote: The Campaign for Emotional

Literacy have their roots in concern about the conditions of life for children and their parents at the beginning of this new millennium.

There is considerable evidence that parents are finding the emotional, as well as the physical, demands of the parenting task hard to balance with the struggle to maintain their roles in the workplace and as partners. It takes time and patience to nurture children and set limits for their behaviour. Finding the quiet space to do this can seem impossible with the increasing demands and pace of modern life. The family is undoubtedly in a time of transition which brings with it feelings of confusion, uncertainty and doubt. Many parents feel adrift, having left behind old certainties about jobs and gender roles but without new, clear values to put in their place. Time to talk about feelings is often sacrificed to pragmatic and practical pressures but children brought up without a language for how they feel are more prone to 'act out' rather than 'speak out'.

Daniel Goleman, in his book *Emotional Intelligence* (1996), believes there is a remedy for this in how we prepare young people for life. At present, he notes that we leave the emotional education of children to chance. Goleman believes that education for being a parent is important to show children that understanding emotional development is not being 'soft' but is a vital component in making and sustaining relationships at home, at school and, increasingly importantly, in the workplace.

Further contemporary evidence of the need for parenting education as a way of improving the quality of emotional relationships between parents and children comes from the recent focus on brain development and function, made possible by advances in brain imaging technology. Howell & Montuschi's article 'Teaching future parents' (1999) notes that emotional impoverishment has long been known as a risk factor for poor educational attainment and social adjustment. What is only now being recognised is that brain development and function are fundamentally affected by the quality of emotional responses in a child's earliest years. In Greenspan's book *The Growth of the Mind and the Endangered Origins of Intelligence* (1996), the eminent American child psychiatrist quotes studies which show that meeting a child's needs for affection and nurturing in a secure, predictable environment helps the brain to make specific neural connections. This in turn affects the development of subtle qualities, such as the ability to engage empathetically with others, to picture another person's intentions and to tolerate ambivalent feelings.

If what is being revealed by the new understanding of the way neural connections are influenced by emotional environment is right, and the links between this and what was already known from developmental psychology suggest that it is, then effective parenting (and high-quality childcare) is likely to be one of *the* vital tasks for the 21st century.

PARENTHOOD EDUCATION IN SCHOOLS: TOO MUCH TOO SOON?

Until quite recently, many experts in the field of child and family development believed parenting education prior to having a child was both suspect and inappropriate. Suspect because of a possibly politically motivated agenda which might promote a particular type of family and inappropriate because it was thought that parenting was the last thing teenagers had on their minds. However, evidence from researchers and writers like Daniel Goleman suggests that, approached in a way which engages the interest of adolescents, education for relationships and parenting may be a popular curriculum subject. This indication is backed by the many organisations which campaign for education which is based on respect, emotional literacy and the promotion of high self-esteem, plus the practical success of the Manchester pilot project. It is evidence such as this, plus the recognition of the impact of parent/child relationships for future social and emotional functioning, which is convincing those in power in the education world that the fundamental components of parenting education should be implicit over all key stages and explicit at Key Stages 3 and 4.

In Toronto, Canada, a programme called Roots of Empathy is currently being taught to children between the ages of four and 14 in over 40 schools. In this programme, which has separate curricula for the different age groups, implicit and explicit components of parenting are shared with small groups of children around the central focus of a 'class baby' who is brought into school by a parent over the infant's first year of life. The children have a chance to follow the progress of 'their' baby and through their curiosity and fascination with the changes that have taken place each time the baby comes, learn about human development, feelings, the perspective of others, the role of the parent and just how time consuming and demanding caring for a baby is. Specialist facilitators from outside the school are trained to help the children address how the baby might be feeling, how the baby's behaviour might make them feel and to make connections with their own behaviour and feelings. (Contact details for this programme, which may be available in the UK soon, are given at the end of the chapter.)

WHAT ABOUT VALUES IN PARENTING EDUCATION?

Both the PASSPORT project (Lees & Plant 2000) and *Two Steps Ahead* (Parenting Education and Support Forum 1998) make a clear case for the values encapsulated in parenting education to permeate the ethos of the school. As Elizabeth Hartley-Brewer puts it in *Two Steps Ahead*:

> It does not make sense for children to be encouraged to listen to others, to respond empathically and to see family life as important at one time in the school day, and then at another to have teachers ignore or deny their state of mind or devalue the impact on them of particular family events. It is, therefore, important for all schools to attend not only to curriculum issues but also those of:

- ethos – respect for individuals, decision-making structures and so on
- pastoral quality and frameworks
- quality partnership with and support for parents
- balance between academic and broader educational goals, such that teachers feel they have permission to give time to respond to family problems that children inevitably bring in to school.

The *Education for Parenthood* (Hope 1998) pack used in the Manchester pilot is rooted in three key principles.

- The uniqueness and potential of every child should be valued.
- Every child should have individual and continuous love and security.
- Parenthood is a privilege and not a right.

The pack also underlines the importance of an approach to delivering parenthood education that specifically avoids overtly or covertly promoting one model of the family as the ideal.

If all pupils are to benefit from parenthood education they must first feel accepted for who they are and the families and cultures they come from. The ethos of parenthood education sessions therefore needs to be accepting and non-judgemental, yet able to offer scope for challenging ill-informed views.

There are, of course, implications here for the selection and training of those who run courses and classes. These issues will be addressed later in the chapter.

BROAD AIMS OF PARENTING EDUCATION IN SCHOOLS

- Expose young people to a way of thinking about parenting as part of the broad spectrum of roles which they are likely to be fulfilling in the future (Howell et al 1997).
- Parenthood education should not tell children what to think or how they should lead their lives when they become parents. It can, however, enable children and young people to learn the *skills* that are necessary to manage family relationships, including marriage; how to sustain relationships; social and communication skills; stress, conflict and time management skills; and how to nurture self-esteem in both children and parents.
- Provide *knowledge* about child development, including the role of play and conversation, how children best learn and children's social, emotional, physical and intellectual needs.
- Develop their *understanding* of some of the reasons for good and bad behaviour and how the parent–child relationship changes; stimulate reflection and discussion of, for example, what the phrase 'good-enough parenting' is trying to convey, what it means in practice and where it might shade into 'not good enough' or even abusive parenting (DfEE 2000, Parenting Education and Support Forum 1998).

WHAT ABOUT SPECIAL NEEDS STUDENTS?

Parenting education seems to be important for special needs students not just because of the content but because they feel they can contribute on an equal level with more able pupils. The experience at Falinge Park High School, which took part in the Manchester pilot and continues to include a 6-week parenting module in its PSHE curriculum for Year 10 students, showed that parenting education supported the self-esteem of less able pupils. One teacher said, 'They had knowledge others might not have'.

BOX 3.4	*Delivering parenthood education*

The *Teacher's Guide to Delivering Parenthood Education* (Sharland & Hope 1998) lists the following examples of ways in which materials can be adapted to suit students of different abilities.

■ Present the instructions on what to do on the chalkboard and talk them through thoroughly rather than copy and hand out the instruction sheets.
■ Use 'student language' rather than 'resource pack jargon' where this is a barrier.
■ Adapt the timings to suit students who work at different speeds.
■ Divide the class up into small groups for discussion.
■ Allow students who are going faster than others to proceed with the next stages in the activity.
■ Use single-sex groupings.
■ Challenge older students about their views and adopt a more discursive and rigorous style of debate.

DOESN'T EDUCATION FOR PARENTHOOD REALLY ONLY APPEAL TO GIRLS?

Evidence from the Manchester pilot of the *Education for Parenthood* (Hope 1998) pack suggests that whilst engaging boys in this topic is more challenging, once involved they can be as committed to the subject as girls. A school nurse quoted in Sharland & Hope (1998) notes: 'Boys who I thought would struggle with this type of information got a lot from the classes because they related it to their own direct experience. Everybody has experience of being parented, don't they?' Students in an all-boys' school in the Manchester pilot demonstrated an enthusiasm for parenthood education and were very comfortable talking about their own experiences and hopes for parenthood amongst their peers and with teachers.

Single-sex groupings can be useful when discussing some aspects of parenthood. Some girls in the pilot project preferred to be on their own when discussing the role of the mother within the home, their approach to working mothers and how to deal with male children, but they said they preferred to be with the boys in other areas of work such as family relationships and handling difficult behaviour as they wanted a male perspective.

Helen Boulter, who coordinates the 6-week parenting modules for Year 10 students as part of a strong PSHE programme at Falinge Park High School in Manchester, believes that mixed-sex groups are appropriate for these sessions. 'Life happens in mixed sex groups', she says, 'so we feel it would be wrong to separate boys and girls to address these issues.'

Sharland & Hope (1998) sum up single-sex and coeducational teaching thus.

■ Teaching male students in all-boys' schools may be more demanding as they show less initial interest in parenthood than female students.

- However, male students in single-sex schools may well respond positively to lessons about parenthood.
- Those in coeducational schools respond in more mature and constructive ways in mixed-sex groupings as the main setting for parenthood delivery.
- Female students in coeducational schools may prefer working in a single-sex group where the male students do not want to take the subject as seriously as they do.
- Female students are often more physically and emotionally mature than male students of the same age. This may be reflected in their interest and the way they respond to discussions about parenthood.

The key to effective and successful teaching of both genders is clearly a skilled and enthusiastic facilitator who has the personal qualities and professional ability to adapt and present materials in ways which are likely to engage the interest of both boys and girls. (See section on Effective Style and Methods for further comment on materials and language suitable to engage boys.)

WHAT DO FACILITATORS NEED IN ORDER TO TEACH EDUCATION FOR PARENTHOOD?

Just as parents need a range of knowledge, skills, understanding and information to undertake their role effectively, so anyone teaching around the subject of parenting needs a range of specialist knowledge, skills and personal qualities (Howell et al 1997). And in parallel to the network of support parents need around them, those teaching this subject need support within the school (if they are teachers or school nurses) as well as from managers and other specialists outside (if they are community-based health professionals).

Hope & Sharland (1997) identified some of the qualities and skills that are required of successful parenthood education facilitators.
Personal qualities:

- warmth
- empathy
- tolerance
- humour
- ability to challenge without undermining
- have high levels of motivation and enthusiasm, and to have chosen to teach the topic
- prepared to discuss matters openly and honestly.

Skills:

- good group work and facilitation skills
- experience of teaching PSHE
- capacity to adapt materials and respond to needs of pupils within sessions.

Teachers participating in the Manchester pilot reported that they had not realised how much there was to consider within the topic of parenthood. Not only was there knowledge content to learn but also, unlike most other subjects, there was an emotional aspect that had an impact on their own personal lives and circumstances. Some teachers remarked that they had modified their own parenting as a result of teaching the course.

Most important of all, Hope & Sharland (1997) recognised the vital importance of factors other than facilitators' enthusiasm, knowledge and skills which had to be in place for parenthood education to be successful in the curriculum of a school. These included:

- an interested and supportive LEA
- supportive school governors
- a committed head teacher
- a secure place in the timetable (the PSHE slot, but with a specific module for parenting education, was found to be most successful in the pilot)
- volunteer teachers with good communication skills and training in group work.

Parenthood and family life education facilitators do not necessarily have to be part of a school's teaching staff. School nurses, who have the mixed benefits of not being part of the school teaching hierarchy but nevertheless are familiar faces in a school and have the opportunity to build relationships with pupils, can be excellent facilitators if they have the appropriate skills and personal qualities.

Health visitors, health education or family planning personnel or even local practice nurses all have roles to play as partners to experienced PSHE teachers. However, bringing in professionals from outside a school to teach parenting classes may not prove beneficial unless the people involved are particularly skilled at communication with young people. The benefit to the ethos of the whole school may also be lost if those coming from outside do not have the time, funding or motivation to get involved in the life of the school.

Not all those who are interested in teaching education for parenthood will have the necessary skills. However, training in counselling skills and group work may be available in house in some Health Authorities or Trusts or there may be money available for training to work in this area through various government initiatives. The Parenting Education and Support Forum is a good source of up-to-date information on training courses and sources of funding for training.

EFFECTIVE STYLES AND METHODS OF WORKING

Teaching about parenting is a process, starting with the underlying or generic understandings and skills in the implicit curriculum of the primary school and being steadily built on as the young person matures and is able to think about the future in secondary school. The PASSPORT project (Lees & Plant 2000) shows how these building blocks can be put in place using the DfEE frameworks and details the learning outcomes at each key stage.

As previously discussed, a didactic style is not appropriate for this subject area. An open, participative style, using experiential techniques and group-work skills, is best.

The language and concepts used should be jargon free and familiar and acceptable to all. Special attention should be paid to the needs of boys as they can easily become alienated or disengaged by subject matter and language which can seem too 'girly' or lead to anti-male bias or banter.

Materials used can be as broad, varied and contemporary as the topic demands. Television 'soaps' often address parenting issues; magazines for both young men and women have letters or articles about young people's experiences with parents; visits can be made to children's centres or visitors invited to the school; surveys and debates can be conducted, job descriptions and games devised and worksheets completed. Materials such as the *Education for Parenthood* pack (Hope 1998) and *Parenting Perspectives* (Howell et al 1997) contain exercises which are linked to key stages. These can be used on their own or supplemented with materials from other sources, up-to-date news clippings, magazine articles, etc.

CONCLUSION

Changes taking place in our society are raising fundamental questions about the nature of motherhood and fatherhood, the balance between work and family life and what constitutes good child rearing and child care. We know more now than ever before that the quality of children's environments and social experience has a decisive, long lasting impact on their development, well being and ability to learn. The decisions – major and mundane – that parents, carers and teachers make every day as they interact with children, help determine whether the children will have the capacity to develop into capable, productive, responsible, emotionally healthy individuals and citizens. (Excerpt from the rationale behind Parent Child 2000, an international 3-day symposium on Early Years Development and Learning, Childcare and Parenting held in London in April 2000, available from Parenting Education and Support Forum.)

The above quote clearly sets out why education for parenting is indeed one of the foremost tasks of the new millennium. Teachers cannot be expected to take on this job alone. School nurses and health professionals working in the local community have a key role to play in partnership with schools and PSHE specialists: health workers sharing the curriculum burden with teachers and schools playing their part in positive preventive health work. Just as parents set the tone and standards for their children's attitudes and behaviour, schools also convey their values through the way both students and staff are treated. Empathic, supportive relationships can only flourish in an atmosphere where there is trust and respect at every level between staff, pupils and all those who contribute to the life of the school. In this ethos children learn their own value and the value of others and can move with confidence towards maturity and making appropriate choices about their lives, including the positive choice of parenthood.

Schools and communities where these values are inherent in everyday practice are pleasant places to work, grow and learn for everybody. Education for parenting has a significant part to play in improving the quality of life for all.

- Interest in education for parenting in schools emerged from concern about teenage pregnancy, family breakdown, aggressive and antisocial behaviour by young people, especially boys.

- The focus on parenting acknowledges, amongst other things, that what goes on between a parent and child in the privacy of their own home has an impact on the capacity of the next generation to take their place as effective citizens and parents.

- All children and young people can benefit from education for parenting, providing the content, style, approach and language are appropriate for the subject matter and the students' stage of development.

- Health professionals as well as specialist PSHE teachers have a vital role to play in both the *implicit* and *explicit* parenting curricula at all key stages.

- Willingness to reflect on one's own parenting (or way of having been parented), flexibility, an ability to feel comfortable with intimate material, excellent communication skills plus group-work training are fundamental requirements for any facilitator of parenting education.

REFERENCES

Department for Education and Employment 1997, Excellence in Schools. HMSO, London

Department for Education and Employment 1999 National Healthy School Standard. Getting started: a guide for schools. DfEE, London

Department for Education and Employment (forthcoming) Parenthood education: guidance for schools. DfEE, London

Goleman D 1996 Emotional intelligence: why it can matter more than IQ. Bloomsbury Publishing, London

Greenspan S 1996 The growth of the mind and the endangered origins of intelligence. Addison Wesley, Reading, Mass

Hope P 1998 Education for Parenthood pack. The Children's Society, London

Hope P, Sharland P 1997 Tomorrow's parents: developing parenthood education in schools. Calouste Gulbenkian Foundation, London

Howell E, Montuschi O 1999 Teaching future parents. Managing Schools Today 8 (8): 9–10

Howell E, Montuschi O, Kahn T 1997 Parenting perspectives: a guide to teaching parenting skills. Courseware Publications, Suffolk

Lees J, Plant S 2000 PASSPORT: a framework for personal and social development. Calouste Gulbenkian Foundation, London

Parenting Education and Support Forum 1998 Two steps ahead: fitting parents for the future. Parenting Education and Support Forum, London

Sharland P, Hope P 1998 Teacher's guide to delivering parenthood education: *The Children's Society*, London

FURTHER READING

Hope P, Sharland P 1997 Tomorrow's parents: developing parenthood education in schools. Calouste Gulbenkian Foundation, London *Excellent report of the pilot project in five Manchester schools using the Education for Parenthood materials. This should be read even if you are not intending to use these particular materials.*

Sharland P, Hope P 1998 Education for parenthood: teacher's guide to delivering parenthood education. The Children's Society, London

This is the accompanying guide to the Education for Parenthood pack, which was piloted in five Manchester schools with young people aged 14–18 years. It is a 'must have' for inexperienced facilitators using the pack, but also of great value to those who want ideas about planning coherent sessions, what sort of exercises go down well and guidance on cultural diversity, gender issues and do's and don'ts in the classroom. There is also an excellent self-assessment questionnaire at the back – Am I ready to teach parenthood?

Lees T, Plant S 2000 PASSPORT: a framework for personal and social development. Calouste Gulbenkian Foundation, London
Building on the DfEE framework for PSHE and Citizenship, PASSPORT identifies the common core of skills, knowledge and understanding, attitudes and values which constitute a pupil's basic entitlement to personal and social development. It also provides comprehensive learning outcomes from Key Stage 1 to Key Stage 4.

Department for Education and Employment (forthcoming) Parenthood education: guidance for schools. DfEE, London
The horse's mouth. Up-to-date, clear guidance on what the parenthood curriculum looks like at each key stage, how to develop modules with practical examples of content and a section on qualities and skills needed by facilitators. Written for the Department by a team of parent education specialists led by Penny Sharland.

Some of the books below are American. Please don't let this put you off. They are excellent, often available in this country or can easily be obtained via the Internet, sometimes at discount prices.

Faber A, Mazlish E 1996 How to talk so kids can learn at home and in school. Fireside Books, USA
All about positive communication.

Murray L, Andrews L 2000 The social baby – understanding babies' communication from birth. CP Publishing, Richmond, Surrey
Wonderfully illustrated book demonstrating how babies communicate from the moment of birth and showing how sensitive caretaking comes about through careful watching and tuning in to the individual baby's communications.

Brazelton TB 1994 Touchpoints: your child's emotional and behavioural development. Perseus Books Group, USA
Touchpoints are critical times in the development of a baby/child. American paediatrician Berry Brazelton helps parents recognise what is going on so that they may better tune in to their child's needs and development.

Lansdown R, Walker M 1996 Your child's development from birth to adolescence. Frances Lincoln, London
Not just about walking and talking but emotional development and needs, too.

Galinsky E 1987 The six stages of parenthood. Addison Wesley, Reading, Mass
This book has never been bettered as an account of how parents' growth and development is led by their children's developmental stages and how parents'

responses need to be attuned to their child's emotional needs and development.

Shore R 1997 Rethinking the brain – new insights into early development. Families and Work Institute, New York
Neuroscience for beginners; how children learn in the context of relationships and how the emotional climate affects how connections in the brain are made and sustained. Very accessible without trivialising the subject.

Campion MJ 1995 Who's fit to be a parent? Routledge, London
There are many contexts in which professionals have to assess adults for their fitness to be parents: when children are taken into care, following divorce, when parents are severely mentally or physically disabled or where medical intervention is necessary in order to conceive a child. This book addresses the difficult questions society has to ask in order for the professionals involved to be able to carry out their roles in an acceptable way.

Golombok S 2000 Parenting: what really counts? Routledge, London
Professor Golombok is Director of the Family and Child Research Centre at City University, London. In this very accessible book she examines the scientific evidence relating to what really matters for children's healthy psychological development.

Hardyment C 1995 Perfect parents: baby-care advice past and present. Oxford University Press, Oxford
How babycare advice for parents has changed over the last century and the influences that have brought about these changes.

Burgess A 1997 Fatherhood reclaimed: the making of the modern father. Vermilion, London
Exploration of modern fatherhood. Draws on interviews with a wide range of fathers as well as excerpts from diaries and biographies.

Gieve K 1989 Balancing acts: on being a mother. Virago, London
Women from different backgrounds and cultures and sexuality give frank accounts of their feelings about and experiences of being a mother.

Lovell A 1995 When your child comes out. Sheldon Press, London
Advice and support for parents and young people in relation to breaking news about sexuality.

Skynner R, Cleese J 1984 Families and how to survive them. Methuen, London
Old it may be, but this book of conversations between family therapist Robin Skynner and funny man John Cleese is still a brilliant way to begin to understand relationships in families.

Tizard B, Phoenix A 1993 Black, white or mixed race? Race and racism in the lives of young people with mixed parentage. Routledge, London
Content as indicated in the title.

Young Minds 1997 Mental health in your school: a guide for teachers and others working in schools. Jessica Kingsley Publications, London
Excellent supportive book for teachers and others working with young people in schools.

RESOURCES

Howell E, Montuschi O, Kahn T 1997 Parenting perspectives: a guide to teaching parenting skills. Courseware Publications, Suffolk
This ring-bound A4 book starts with a chapter on the social and economic reasons behind the current interest in parenting education. The following four sections, entitled 'What Do Parents Do?', 'The Stages of Parenthood', 'Parenting Styles' and 'Culture and Equality Issues' are intended as background reading for teachers and older pupils. The last section contains 30 photocopiable classroom activity sheets linked to the different sections. Symbols indicate appropriateness for key stages and links to the National Curriculum. Activities are aimed at older Key Stage 2 children and above.

Hope P 1998 Education for parenthood: a resource pack for young people. The Children's Society, London
A pack of five booklets containing 28 classroom and community-based activities designed to encourage participative and experiential learning about parenthood. All exercises linked to the National Curriculum. Aimed at Years 9 and 10 upwards.

Tufnell G (ed) 2000 Mental health and growing up: factsheets for parents, teachers and young people. Royal College of Psychiatrists, London
36 facts sheets in A4 pack.

Videos

Getting Through the Day: A Survival Guide for Parents
Carlton TV, PO Box 101, London WC2N 4AW
Everyday scenarios with parents and children under five, showing helpful and not helpful ways of handling children's behaviour.

Teenagers: A Survival Guide for Parents
Carlton TV (as above)
Realistic scenarios between teenagers and their parents which could be helpful in encouraging young people to see parents' perspective.

Both these videos are under £5 and come with an accompanying booklet.

Teenagers in Trouble
Trust for the Study of Adolescence, 23 New Road, Brighton BN1 1W2
Very realistic (including bad language) scenarios between parents and teenagers, plus discussion from group of parenting professionals. Devised for use with parents who have been sent on parenting programmes by the courts, but has great potential for stimulating discussion with teenagers on topic of family relationships. The video comes with a facilitator's guide.

Useful contacts and addresses

Roots of Empathy Programme, 401 Richmond Street West, Suite 205, Toronto, Ontario M5V 3A8, Canada
Tel: (416) 944-3001
Fax: (416) 944-9295
Email: mail@rootsofempathy.org
Website: www.rootsofempathy.org

Parenting Education and Support Forum, 431 Highgate Studios, 53–79 Highgate Road, London NW5 1TL
Tel: 0207 284 8370
Email: pesf@dial.pipex.com
Websites: www.parentingforum.org.uk, www.parenthood.org.uk *(special website for parenting education in schools)*
Promotes parenting education and provides support and information for professionals from all backgrounds.

Antidote: The Campaign for Emotional Literacy, 5th Floor, 45 Beech Street, London EC2Y 8AD
Tel: 0207 588 5151
Email: antidote@geo2.poptel.org.uk
Promotes and supports emotional literacy in schools and all aspects of life.

Child Psychotherapy Trust, Star House, 104–108 Grafton Road, London NW5 4BD
Tel: 0207 284 1355
Fax: 0207 7284 2755
Email: cpt@globalnet.co.uk
Website www.childpsychotherapytrust.org.uk
Promotes public understanding of emotional development of children and significance of relationships between parent and child. Publishes excellent range of leaflets and posters on emotional health and well-being of children.

Jenny Mosley Consultancies, 8 Westbourne Road, Trowbridge, Wiltshire BA14 0AJ
Tel: 01225 767157
Fax: 01225 755631
Email: circletime@jennymosley.demon.co.uk
Website: www.jennymosley.demon.co.uk
Offers consultancy to primary, secondary and special schools wishing to develop Circle Time. Jenny Mosley has written extensively on this subject and is an acknowledged expert.

RELATE in schools
Via local RELATE centres or information from Martin Carr, National Training Director, RELATE, Herbert Gray College, Little Church Street, Rugby, Warwickshire CV21 3AP
Tel: 01788 573241
Website: www.relate.org.uk
Runs courses to equip teachers and others with the confidence and classroom techniques demanded by the issues dealt with in relationship education, as well as specialist subject workshops.

Young Minds, 102–108 Clerkenwell Road, London EC1M 5SA
Tel: 0207 336 8445
Fax: 0207 336 8446
Email: enquiries@youngminds.org.uk
Website: www.youngminds.org.uk
Parents/professionals information service: 0800 018 2138. Available for anyone with concerns about the mental health of a young person/people. Young Minds also has a training and consultancy service.

Parenting Connections Consultancy (Elizabeth Howell), 14 Somali Road, London NW2 3RL
Tel: 0207 813 9190
Email: howell01@globalnet.co.uk
Consultancy and training for all those concerned with education for parenting. Also has extensive library of parenting programmes for use with parents and books and videos on all aspects of child development and parenting.

Specialist publishers

The Children's Society, Edward Rudolf House, Margery Street, London WC1X 0JL
Tel: 0207 841 4400
Email: publishing@childsoc.org.uk

Calouste Gulbenkian Foundation, 98 Portland Place, London W1N 4ET
Tel: 0207 636 5313

Courseware Publications, 4 Apple Barn Court, Westley, Suffolk IP33 3TJ
Tel/Fax: 01284 703300
Email: courseware@btinternet.com

Department for Education and Employment Publications, PO Box 5050, Annesley, Nottingham NG15 0DJ
Tel: 0845 6022260
Fax: 0845 6055560
Email: dfee@prologistics.co.uk
Or visit the Wired for Health website at www.wiredforhealth.gov.uk

Trust for the Study of Adolescence, 23 New Road, Brighton BN1 1WZ
Tel: 01273 693311
Fax: 01273 679907
Email: publications@tsa.uk.com
Website: www.tsa.uk.com

4 Parent partnership

Sue White

INTRODUCTION

Professionals in the fields of health and social care will be aware that the concept of working in partnership with parents has been a topic of conversation for many years. Many of those professionals will have felt constrained, by a variety of factors, from putting partnership working into practice; others will have felt that they lacked confidence or information about how partnership could or should be put into practice. A further group may reluctantly admit that they are unsure about the concept of partnership, how it is defined and what it 'looks like' in practice.

This chapter aims to:

■ clarify the parent partnership concept
■ put forward a model for working in partnership with parents
■ look at the issues that may be holding professionals back from this way of working
■ suggest ways in which these issues may be overcome.

WHAT DO WE MEAN BY 'WORKING IN PARTNERSHIP WITH PARENTS'?

There are many interpretations of the term 'parent partnership' and perhaps this is why it is so difficult for us to grasp its meaning. In my experience, responses to the question 'What is parent partnership?' usually fall into one of the following categories.

■ It's respecting parents.
■ It's about professionals working with parents.
■ It's giving parents a say.
■ It's difficult to do, but it's about involving parents in everything to do with service provision to their family.
■ It's giving parents information.
■ I'm not too sure, but we are being asked to do it these days, especially if we are seeking grant funding.

I believe that in many ways parent partnership encompasses all these and more. However, it is important that the concept is clarified, so that appropriate goals may be set by organisations and individual professionals, regarding the process of developing this way of working.

Several definitions of parent partnership have been proposed. For example, it was suggested as far back as 1983 that partnership involves:

> . . . a full sharing of knowledge, skills and experiences . . . partnership can take many forms, but it must by definition be on a basis of equality, in which each side has areas of knowledge and skills that it contributes to the joint task of working with the child. (Mittler & Mittler 1983:10–11).

Around the same time, Wolfendale (1983) suggested that partnership involved 'equivalent expertise'. These ideas were expanded in a frequently cited definition proposed by Pugh & De'Ath (1989) a few years later. They suggested that partnership is: 'a working relationship that is characterised by a shared sense of purpose, mutual respect and the willingness to negotiate. This implies a sharing of information, responsibility, skills, decision making and accountability' (p. 68).

The key ideas contained in definitions of partnership working may be summed up in the following.

- Equality
- Equivalent expertise
- Sharing knowledge
- Sharing skills
- Sharing experience
- Sharing information
- Sharing responsibility
- Sharing accountability
- Joint purpose
- Mutual respect
- Negotiation.

Professionals work in many ways in relation to their service users. In order to examine these different ways, many models of working have been discussed and a resumé of the main ones follows. Looking at these will help to further clarify what is meant by the phrase 'working in partnership with parents'.

THE EXPERT MODEL

In this way of working, an example of which is the traditional doctor/patient relationship, the professional:

- is seen as the expert
- assumes that it is his or her responsibility to solve the parent's problems
- takes control
- makes judgements about what needs doing
- does not necessarily seek the views and feelings of the parent.

The parent:

- provides information
- is expected to comply with advice
- is not part of the decision-making process.

The advantages of the expert model are:

- the professional's skills are fully used
- the burden of decision making and responsibility is removed from the parent.

The disadvantages are:

- the parent feels powerless and inferior
- the parent feels excluded from decisions
- the aspirations of the professional and parent may be different
- the professional may give inappropriate information which the parent may not wish or be able to take.

THE TRANSPLANT MODEL

In this model, described by Dorothy Jeffree in the 1970s and cited by Mittler & Mittler (1983), the professional is willing to involve the parent more.
The professional:

- shares, or transplants, his or her expertise and skills in order to help parents increase their skills
- helps the parents become actively involved in the work with their own child
- sees the parents as a resource with particular abilities which can be used
- retains the power
- retains final control in decision making.

The parents:

- are expected to become involved
- gain skills
- gain confidence.

The advantages of the transplant model are:

- professionals need to examine, and make changes to, their practice
- professionals need to communicate with parents
- professionals have to develop new skills which will enable them to transfer their knowledge to parents
- parents are more involved
- parents develop new skills.

The disadvantages are:

- not all parents are ready and willing to get involved
- parents are dependent upon the professionals' skills and expertise
- parents can become less confident in their own ability as the professionals are still seen as the experts in the relationship
- the professionals retain the power in the relationship.

THE CONSUMER MODEL

In this model, described by Cunningham & Davis (1985), the parent is seen as the 'purchaser' of services and, as such, has choice and some power.

The professional:

- is seen as guiding the parent
- assists the parent in making appropriate decisions
- communicates and negotiates with the parent.

The parent:

- has power over access to resources
- has the right to select services that are appropriate to his or her needs and can opt in or out of service provision
- is seen as having skills and knowledge that are distinct from those of the professional. The professional acknowledges that the parent 'knows' his or her own child
- the parent has the opportunity to challenge the professional's position.

The advantages of working in this way are:

- the intervention is tailored to the individual family
- professionals need to critically analyse their service delivery
- parents are placed in a more powerful position
- parents' skills are developed and their power acknowledged.

The disadvantages are:

- the model assumes that all parents are ready and able to negotiate on their own and their family's behalf
- it assumes that parents know what they need and how to find it
- in reality, budget restrictions limit service user power and choice
- it develops partnership with individuals rather than with whole user groups.

THE EMPOWERMENT MODEL

This model, described in 1991 by Appleton & Minchom, recognises the individuality of families and the need for professionals to work to empower parents, rather than allowing them to become dependent on professional support.
The professional:

- recognises the parent's right to choose the degree to which he or she becomes involved with the service
- needs to consider what help the parent needs in order to be empowered
- needs to help the parent to become a partner in service delivery
- encourages the parent to take control and make decisions.

The parent:

- chooses his or her own level of involvement
- takes greater responsibility for decision making
- develops greater confidence and power as a result of the intervention.

The advantages of the empowerment model are:

- it emphasises the need for professionals to help parents to take control
- it recognises diversity of service users

- it builds on existing strengths and skills and develops new ones.

The disadvantage is that:

- the parents may not wish to be equal partners.

THE NEGOTIATOR MODEL

This model was proposed by Dale in 1996 and uses the following definition of partnership:

> . . . a working relationship where the partners use negotiation and joint decision-making and resolve differences of opinion and disagreement, in order to reach some kind of shared perspective or jointly agreed decision on issues of mutual concern. (p. 14)

Dale describes the negotiator model as having several key elements:

- the parent and professional have separate and valuable contributions to make, but they come to the encounter with different perspectives
- the professional has a responsibility to strive to bridge the gap between the various perspectives
- the professional may adopt the role of expert, instructor, consultant or facilitator but these role options must be negotiated with the parent.

Dale points out that 'transactions in a partnership relationship may be a cyclical process which shifts back and forth between agreement and disagreement' (p. 5). The model acknowledges that sometimes there is a conflict in the relationship which cannot be resolved and the partnership may temporarily or permanently break down.

Advantages of the negotiator model are that:

- it recognises the differing experiences and perspectives of the parent and the professional
- it acknowledges that conflict situations arise
- it places a responsibility upon the professional to make changes to practice to enable a partnership relationship to develop.

The disadvantages of the model are:

- the professional retains the power
- it does not assume that, on occasions, the parent will take the lead in the development of the partnership
- it does not provide a solution in situations where the partnership breaks down
- the breakdown of the partnership can be devastating and 'disempowering' for professionals and parents.

An examination of the above models moves the professional from total control, as in the expert model, toward an 'equivalent expertise' and negotiation situation and it is this shift that is central for an organisation or professional wishing to move toward partnership working.

Rather than accept or dispense with any of these models per se, I would suggest that what is required in true partnership working is a combination of them. Since partnership must be dynamic and flexible in order to meet the changing needs of parents and the organisation, I see parent partnership as follows:

> *A relationship between an organisation providing services to parents and those parents who use the services. In this relationship, the planning, development, delivery and monitoring of services are shared at all times and in every respect. There will be occasions when one or other partner takes the lead for a period of time but this partner will not assume power and the balance will be redressed when the other partner is ready. There is an implicit understanding of differing but equivalent roles and expertise and negotiation and compromise are viewed as integral to the relationship, as are respect, trust, openness and choice.*

I would maintain that the above view takes into account the following example situations that are encountered by every service.

When a parent is first introduced to a service, that parent may not wish to become involved in the way in which it is delivered. She may choose to receive the service in the traditional way. It is this right of choice that is important in relation to parent partnership. Urgent situations arise which force the service providers to make decisions without calling together a representative group of parents. This is one occasion where the professionals take the lead for a period of time, but because of the trust and openness that have been built up with parents, the situation is understood by parents. They know that they have not been excluded and that they will be informed fully about the decisions that have been taken and why. In child protection situations, while every effort should be made to work in partnership with parents, if the service provider considers that a child will be placed at greater risk if parents are involved in discussions, the provider must take the appropriate action and forego partnership working. It is vital, however, that the balance is redressed as soon as possible and that every effort is made to regain a partnership relationship.

Some definitions of partnership working have now been explored and various models have been discussed to help to clarify the concept. We will now examine it at a practical level.

WHAT COULD PARTNERSHIP WITH PARENTS LOOK LIKE?

It may be helpful to look at this from:

- the parents' perspective
- the healthcare team's perspective
- the individual professional's perspective.

The parents' perspective

The healthcare team values the parents and acknowledges their experience, skills and culture. The parents feel confident in all their dealings with the team. They feel that the team has their best interests at heart and they are aware of all the policies of the team. The parents trust the team to be open and honest at all times and know that no action will be taken without their prior permission (except regarding issues of child protection). The parents' skills, confidence and self-esteem are enhanced through contact with the team.

The healthcare team's perspective

The team has a policy on working in partnership with parents and has regular discussions and training sessions relating to partnership. Supervision sessions and staff meetings provide good opportunities for these types of discussion. Parents are involved collectively in all major decisions regarding the team's relationship with parents and individually in all decisions regarding their own family. The team includes parents as *equal* partners, e.g. as volunteers, as trainers and speakers. All written information about a family, while confidential, is available to that family. This, again, may not be possible in child protection situations but parents should be made aware of this from the first encounter with the team. Parents are fully involved in all evaluations of the healthcare team's services to parents. This includes involvement at the evaluation planning stage and, if questionnaires are to be used, parents are involved in the design and piloting of the questionnaires.

The individual professional's perspective

The professional shares all information with the parent. This includes all information relevant to that particular family and all relevant information about the healthcare team. The professional invites the parent to become part of the team's service planning and delivery mechanism. The professional respects and values the parent's skills, time, experience and culture and involves the parent in all decisions relating to her family. Permission is obtained from the parent prior to any discussion about the family with any other professional or individual. This includes internal discussions within the team. The professional shares her knowledge and skills with the parent and is open and honest with the parent about the limitations of that knowledge.

The above examples are intended to give the reader a flavour of parent partnership working, but what are the advantages and challenges to all parties in working in this way?

WHY WORK IN PARTNERSHIP WITH PARENTS?

In recent years, the move toward working in partnership with parents has been encouraged by government legislation, e.g. the Children Act (1989) and the Education Act (1993). Indeed, some recent initiatives have insisted that parent partnership is an integral part of service development and delivery and availability of funding has, in part, been dependent upon it, e.g. SureStart, New Deal for Communities.
In this section I explore:

- the benefits of working in partnership
- challenges and barriers to this way of working.

I have included the points that most professionals raise in discussions on the topic.

There are many benefits of working in partnership with parents. First, the combined effort of parent and professional means that extra skills are available to both. Partnership working encourages and fosters openness between service provider and service user and values people and the skills and experience they have. Working in partnership with parents dilutes the barriers that often exist between service providers and service users and community involvement raises cultural awareness. Parental involvement saves the professional time in the longer term. Initially the professional may need to spend extra time assisting the parent to be involved, but once this is done the benefits will be obvious. Services that are designed and developed in partnership will be more relevant to service users' needs and the parent and professional will work toward shared goals and develop a shared understanding of the service's capabilities and its limitations. They will also share challenges and often a parent will find a solution to a problem that the professional (bound by the needs of the workplace and not necessarily part of the local community) would not be able to provide.

Partnership working is satisfying for both professionals and service users, because goals, experiences, ideas, problem solving and celebrations of success are shared. It is very empowering for parents to be 'taken on' by professionals as equal partners. It is also empowering for professionals to know that they have been instrumental in developing parents' skills and experience. And since mutual respect is an integral part of working in partnership, both parents and professionals feel that their views have been listened to.

On the other hand, there are challenges and barriers to working in partnership with parents. First, professionals sometimes find the idea of working in partnership with parents threatening. They may fear a loss of control and that it may erode their hard-earned professional status. They worry about exposure of their limitations and the blurring of the boundary lines between the parent and professional. In practice, the boundaries are maintained when the professional and parent remember the purpose of the relationship. Some professionals also worry about the competence of service users, their commitment levels and their accountability. I believe that it is the responsibility of professionals to give parents sufficient information and training to ensure that these concerns are overcome. Apathy can be a barrier to partnership working. For example, if parents are not interested in working in partnership or if they are too busy or suffer with depression, it may be difficult to engage them. Particularly in the early stages, it may not be possible to engage with a range of users but professionals should not make this an excuse for dispensing with partnership working, as once the practice is developed, it will gather its own momentum and more parents will want to become involved.

Professionals often cite the 'hard-to-reach families' as a reason for not working in partnership. As I have stated previously, I do not believe that families are 'hard to reach', I believe that services are hard to reach and that we need to find ways to make them more accessible to our potential service users. An ethos of working in partnership is a good starting point.

Partnership working can take more of the professional's time, especially in the early stages. It is much easier to go ahead and plan services in staff meetings without going to the trouble of involving parents who may take longer to make decisions, may need to meet at different times, may have training needs and may want to dispute the professionals' views! Furthermore, professionals enjoy the use of jargon, abbreviations and 'buzz words'. Working in partnership means that the jargon has to be dropped. Confidentiality can become an issue in partnership working and this will need to be looked at carefully. A confidentiality policy may need to be written or the current policy modified. There could be cost implications to working in partnership with parents (but there may also be cost savings).

Professionals fear that parents who are involved in the development and monitoring of service provision will come with their own agenda and vested interests and that they will not be able to take an overview of the needs of the majority of service users. Professionals also fear that they will not be able to meet the conflicting demands of a range of parents. These fears are understandable but with respect, negotiation and compromise at the heart of partnership, my experience does not show these issues to be insurmountable.

It is fair to say, however, that a professional in a large multidisciplinary team who wants to work in partnership faces an uphill struggle if the team does not follow the same agenda. In this situation, the professional concerned will need to raise awareness first with immediate colleagues. Following this, an approach can be made to senior colleagues to suggest steps toward partnership working. The lack of precedent may be a barrier that needs to be overcome.

MOVING TOWARDS WORKING IN PARTNERSHIP WITH PARENTS

There are two main factors that will decide whether your team moves forward on this issue or not.

- A sincere willingness to work in partnership with parents.
- An understanding of what is meant by partnership working.

A sincere willingness to work in partnership with parents

You may think that this is obvious, that you wouldn't be reading this if you were not sincere and willing to work in this way. But remember the challenges that were discussed earlier. Apply them honestly to yourself and to your colleagues and the people who drive policy and practice within your team.

 If partnership working is to be developed, everyone will need to become committed to it.

Members of the team will need to be prepared to gain a shared understanding of the concept, be convinced of its merits and be willing to work towards its development at all times. This is not to say that individuals cannot make a difference. The individual professional can work in partnership with parents with whom she comes into contact but it will not be possible to involve the parents in decision-making processes if this is not the team policy.

An understanding of what is meant by partnership working

Your team will need to explore the meaning of working in partnership with parents and to envisage how this will change policy and practice. What better way to begin the process than to invite some parents who use your services to join in with this process of exploration? A common mistake is to feel that you need to have all the answers before parents are involved. You may fear appearing weak or lacking in some way in front of service users. Remember, we are all human. We all have skills and expertise but we have different skills and expertise and limits to our knowledge. It is not essential for you to have all the answers.

Assuming, now, that your team is committed to working in partnership with parents, many questions begin to present themselves.

What is important in partnership working is for professionals and service users to find the answers *together*.

- What policy changes will your team need to make?
- How does your team go about making changes to practice?
- What skills will you have to acquire?
- What skills will parents need to acquire?
- How do you access parents?

These questions form the starting point for exploring how you can move toward working in partnership with parents now that your team has shared, developed and communicated a vision of the meaning of partnership.

WHAT POLICY CHANGES WILL YOU NEED TO MAKE?

Clearly, if you have not been working in partnership with parents before now, you will need to examine all your policies and make changes to reflect the philosophy of partnership. I would suggest that it is vital at this stage to involve parents in the whole process of examining policies and developing new ones. If parents are not involved:

- the team is not serious about partnership
- you cannot expect parents to be happy with policies that have been developed by professionals alone.

The number and type of necessary changes will, of course, depend on the current practice of your team. Table 4.1 may help to identify the starting point for your particular team and assist in planning the next steps.

Note that each stage builds on the previous stage. This is not meant to be a definitive list but to be used as a guide to the stage your team has reached in partnership working. There should be enough detail in each category to allow you to assess progress and to give guidance as to the changes necessary in order to move onto the next stage. You will not necessarily move from one stage to another in all categories at the same time, although once the partnership ethos has been fully understood and accepted by the team as a whole, the transition from Stage One to Stage Four could happen relatively quickly.

TABLE 4.1	*Stages in the development of parent partnership working*			
	Stage One	**Stage Two**	**Stage Three**	**Stage Four**
General philosophy of the team	Team has discussed PPW. General recognition that this would be helpful. Parents involved in the service provision to their children.	Specific meetings are held to discuss PPW. Parents are involved in some way (other than as service receivers).	Mission statement refers to parent partnership. The mission statement was written in partnership with parents.	Team monitors partnership activity and reports about the effectiveness of its work. Staff appraisals and supervision sessions contain discussion about PPW. Parents are involved at all levels.
Recruitment	Staff recruited for new services to parents.	Parents are informed about new staff recruitment and invited to meet new personnel.	Parents discuss with you the proposals to recruit new staff. Parents are involved in writing of job descriptions, job adverts.	Parents are involved as equal partners with staff in all aspects of recruitment, including the assessment of applications, shortlisting, interviews, induction programme.
Service development	Team and managers design new services and changes to existing provision.	Team and management design new services and ask parents for their views on the design.	Parents are consulted before a new service is designed or a current service is changed. Parents are involved in service development.	Parents are consulted at all stages of designing a new service. Parents are involved as equal partners in design of all new services for parents or changes to existing ones.
Service monitoring and evaluation	Healthcare team monitors and evaluates service provision and uptake.	Parents are asked on a regular basis to comment on service provision (usually on a questionnaire or at a focus group, etc.).	Parents are involved on service monitoring groups.	Parents are involved as equal partners with healthcare team in all aspects of monitoring and evaluation, including the design of questionnaires, briefing of research consultants, receiving full reports on monitoring.

(cont'd)

Stages in the development of parent partnership working (cont.)

Training	Stage One	Stage Two	Stage Three	Stage Four
	Training is provided for healthcare team. Training is designed and delivered by team.	Training is provided for parents and team.	Identical training is provided for team and parents; they attend joint training.	Training is designed and delivered by team and parents, to team and parents.
Staff team	The healthcare team meets on a regular basis.	The team welcomes parents into its building or office space, even if no appointment has been made.	The team invites parents into meetings occasionally. The whole team shares some of its social activities with parents.	The team involves service users in some meetings and activities and social activities. Whenever a meeting is planned, thought is given to inviting parents.
Service provision	The team makes all the decisions about service provision.	Parents have the opportunity to choose which services they require.	Parents are consulted individually to find out when, and how, they wish to receive the service.	Parents are involved in the provision of the service to other parents. Parents are involved in the design of all service provision.
Policies of the organisation	The healthcare team writes and agrees all the policies.	The policies are made available to parents. Parents are consulted when new policies are written.	Parents are automatically offered copies of the policies. Parents are included in the writing of new policies.	Parents are included as equal partners in the writing or amending of policies. All policies reflect and describe PPW.
Written information	Written internal information, e.g. meeting minutes, forward plans, policies, are circulated to healthcare team only.	Written information is available to parents, on request.	All written information about a family is shown to that family as a matter of course. The internal written information of the team is available for parents to read.	The family holds written records about themselves if they wish. Meeting minutes, etc. are circulated to parents who attend the meetings and to other parents if they wish. Meeting minutes are displayed openly at the health centre.

It is important that working in partnership with parents is seen as a process, part of the ongoing development of the team. Looking at Table 4.1, you may assess your team as being at Stage One (or not yet at Stage One). Reaching Stage Four (or beyond) will take many months and possibly years, depending on a variety of factors including:

- the size of the team
- the general attitude of team members
- the complexity of the team and its systems
- the team's change management ability
- the numbers of parents willing to participate in bringing about change.

Remember, working in partnership with parents is a process. You may never arrive at a point where you can say you have totally achieved it. If you do arrive at that point, it may be only temporarily. It is important, however, to keep monitoring the team's progress toward partnership and the progress of the individuals within the team.

HOW DO YOU GO ABOUT MAKING CHANGES TO PRACTICE?

Naturally, practice should follow from policy. Once parents have been involved in developing policies for your team, these parents (and others) need to be included on steering and monitoring groups to ensure that policy and practice are compatible.

The most important thing about making changes to practice is to get started! It will not always be easy and sometimes you will get it wrong. But trying to cover every eventuality in a theoretical way will not ensure perfection in practice. Get out there and do it! Learn with the parents. Don't always feel you have to be a step ahead of them.

WHAT SKILLS WILL PROFESSIONALS NEED TO ACQUIRE?

In my opinion, working in partnership with parents does not require any special skill on the part of the professionals concerned. What will make a difference is a change in attitude. You will need to:

- be determined to work in partnership
- be prepared to give away your knowledge, skills and expertise
- give up the use of professional jargon, abbreviations and 'buzz words'
- be flexible in your working times and patterns (for example, meetings with groups of parents will probably need to take place during school hours and not over the lunch period when parents will want to be at home to feed young children).

You need not fear the loss of your professionalism or your power. Working in partnership and being able to pass on skills is a very empowering experience for all concerned. Parents welcome the openness and honesty of professionals who work in this way. They understand that boundaries remain and that professionals bring an overview and expertise to the situation.

WHAT SKILLS WILL PARENTS NEED TO ACQUIRE?

The major difficulty for parents invited to work in partnership is that they see health professionals as service providers and, historically, parents have not been invited to participate. This history has disempowered parents and made them feel unable to make a valuable contribution. It has not allowed them to assert themselves and has put them in an inferior position in relation to the professionals who deliver the service. When given the choice, parents who bring this history will opt to receive services in the traditional way. It is up to you at this stage to lead the parents and help them adjust to the partnership.

At the beginning of the process, parents will need you to take the lead. Then, if you are seen to be committed to partnership, the parents will soon gain in confidence and feel able to participate fully and equally.

Once parents feel comfortable with the idea of working in partnership with the team providing services, they will embrace the idea wholeheartedly and the process of development, of both the parents and the team, can move forward.

Just as professionals generally have a desire to improve their skill levels in relation to the work they are doing, so parents will want to develop skills to enable them to work with you. Naturally, it is not possible to dictate what these skills will be as they depend on the previous experience of the parents concerned. What is clear, however, is that parents will usually be able to identify their own training needs, once they are aware of the demands of the job that needs to be done.

Some of the more frequently requested training needs are:

- meetings skills
- minute and note taking
- time management
- assertiveness skills
- financial record keeping and budgetary management.

Do these also sound like the type of training courses that you and your colleagues want to attend? If so, bear in mind that joint parent/professional training is a significant measure of working in partnership with parents.

Some other aspects to bear in mind in relation to parents' needs are:

- the provision of crèche facilities to enable parents to attend meetings, etc.
- provision for parents with disabilities. Ensure that meetings are held in accessible buildings. Provide ramps, hearing loops and signing, taped minutes, etc., where necessary
- interpreting services
- arranging meetings to fit in with school hours, young children's eating and sleeping times
- the avoidance of the use of jargon.

And remember that any time that parents give to you and your team to enable you to work in partnership is given on a voluntary basis. *They* don't have to be there.

HOW DO YOU ACCESS PARENTS?

Why do professionals always ask this question? Why do they talk about 'hard-to-reach' families?

When service provision is appropriate to a family's needs, the family will present itself. Don't ask how to get hold of the 'hard-to-reach' family; ask: 'What is it about our service that makes it difficult for some parents to access it?'

Naturally, the only people who can answer this question are the parents who are not currently accessing the service. So how do you find out? Some options for your team to consider are given below. The ability to take up the options will, in part, depend on resources.

- Using an independent researcher to gain the views of families who do not currently use the service.
- Training parents from the local community to gain the views of other parents.
- Obtaining the views of other professionals who *do* work with the families who are not yet accessing your service.
- Setting up a confidential telephone helpline for a week or two to consult with families in the community.

BOX 4.1	*Steps in moving your team towards working in partnership with parents*
	- Step One: the team makes a sincere decision to work in partnership with parents. - Step Two: the team clarifies, together with parents, what is meant by partnership working. - Step Three: the team works out an action plan, together with service users, for moving forward. The action plan will take into account any policy changes, training and research that need to be arranged.

EXAMPLES OF PARENT PARTNERSHIP IN ACTION

Translating theory into practice is rarely straightforward but the two examples that follow describe how partnership with parents has been achieved in two projects. I have focused on both situations where partnership has been difficult and situations where it has developed more easily.

The first example is KIDS, a small national voluntary organisation, providing services for children with disabilities, which I had the privilege of working with for 10 years. My role was to set up services in the North Birmingham area. When I joined, KIDS had services in London and Hull. I describe development in the early years, setting up a family centre in Birmingham.

The second example, the Chinnbrook Children and Parents' Project, provides services for young children in the Billesley area of Birmingham. My involvement was linked with the development of a SureStart programme for Billesley. I describe the project and my impressions of it.

KIDS

KIDS, which has been developing since the early 1970s, provides services which are tailored to meet local need. Its mission statement is as follows.

> Through working in partnership with parents and collaborating with others, KIDS seeks to enable children with disabilities throughout England to develop their skills and abilities, and to fulfil their potential, hopes and aspirations.

In 1989, a funding partnership was agreed between KIDS and the Birmingham Local Education Authority for the development of a Portage service in the North Birmingham area, this being the only area of the city that did not have such a service. Portage is a preschool, home teaching service for children with learning disabilities. The Portage worker visits on a weekly basis and works in partnership with the family to help them to teach their child. The family is then asked to carry out daily activities with the child and monitor the progress made until the Portage worker visits the following week.

The next step was to set up a parents' support group, to reduce the isolation felt by families. The group met at the Portage worker's office – not terribly suitable for children! – and this presented the opportunity for parents to get involved in wider issues regarding service delivery, monitoring and development. Diverting a funding crisis two years later had the effect of bringing the group of parents and the staff (now myself and an administrator) closer together.

As the group of parents receiving Portage enlarged and as they became more aware of KIDS as a national organisation, the desire for a Family Centre providing a range of services, similar to those enjoyed by KIDS' families in London and Hull, grew. For the next five years, some of the parents, together with KIDS Birmingham staff and an educational psychologist from the North Birmingham Educational Psychology team, worked towards the achievement of the Family Centre. This development group worked as a team. A large amount of money had to be raised. Parents shared presentations to potential funders with the paid staff, met the architects and designed the building refurbishment. Parents chose the most suitable building to house the Centre. Parents decided what new services were needed and in which order. In effect, staff provided coordination and administrative back-up.

Finally, the move to the Centre proved to be rather an anticlimax and families feared that they would lose the close family atmosphere that had grown up around the development of the Centre. Staff at this point had to take the lead. They had to encourage the parents to stay involved and to allow other families to become involved. They had to take an overview. Sometimes families' enthusiasm for developing new services, now that there was so much space, overtook the ability to raise funds to support the new services. Staff had to moderate this enthusiasm and present the wider and more long-term view.

These difficulties were shortlived. The new Centre, its staff and service users settled to a changed status quo. A Centre management committee was set up. The members of this committee were parents using the services and staff, who provided reports and advice when requested and serviced the committee. Revised systems were put in place to deal with the rapidly developing Centre and this included the development of policies, which were all debated, amended and agreed by the management committee. In time, service development groups were set up to develop and monitor individual services; the members of these groups were always parents working with the member of staff responsible for the particular service.

The partnership between staff and service users had the effect of empowering the parents. Generally speaking, parents were very vulnerable when they were first referred to KIDS. Their confidence levels were low and they were often reluctant to participate in community activities now that they had a child with a disability. Staff at the Centre 'wrapped the parents in layers of cotton wool and gradually unwrapped the layers' as the parents grew in confidence and the knowledge that they could deal with their situation, albeit with support, and could often help others to do the same. Without the support of the parents, the staff would not have achieved the development of the Centre and its services. If services had been developed, they might not have been appropriate to families' needs. Both parents and staff gained a great deal of satisfaction, knowing that they had set goals together and, despite difficulties, had achieved the goals – together.

The Chinnbrook Children and Parents' Project, Birmingham

In 1994, a multi-agency group working in the Billesley area of Birmingham identified the need for services for preschool children and their parents. The multi-agency group consisted of local parents, schools' personnel, GPs, health visitors, the Community Development Officer, the local councillor and a representative of Leisure and Community Services. It was decided that Leisure and Community Services would manage a new project to be set up to meet the identified needs. A building in the area, owned by Leisure and Community Services, had space available. A successful grant application to the health authority enabled some refurbishment of the building and the employment of two members of staff.

The project coordinator had early years and community development skills and she was supported in her role by a nursery nurse. They began work early in 1996. Their first step was to conduct a community consultation exercise to gain up-to-date information about the specific service requirements of local parents and their young children. The outcome was the development of a parent and toddler group, which was immediately popular and which is still running. This is in contrast to several other groups in the area, started around the same time, which no longer operate.

The stated aim of the project in the Annual Report 1999–2000 is to 'work in partnership with local parents/carers and their preschool children in order to provide preventative, informal services which meet their health and social needs'. Partnership is central to all the work of the Chinnbrook Project and is reflected on a number of different levels. It is evident in ongoing consultation about the services and the way the services are run, in the decision and policy-making processes, in management, fundraising and service delivery. It features clearly in skill, knowledge and information sharing on a day-to-day basis. Partnership with other professionals working in the area enables the project to offer a more consistent and coordinated approach to local families.

Currently the project's programme includes a playgroup, various parent and toddler groups, training courses and support groups for parents, family outings and events and a summer playscheme. The staff team has grown and there is also a team of volunteers recruited by the project. Many of the volunteers are parents who have used or are still using the services at Chinnbrook.

Feedback from families indicates that there are a number of practical outcomes for parents and carers from being involved with the project. These include increased confidence and self-esteem, development of parenting skills, improved family functioning, awareness of other resources/activities within the local area, development of friendship and support networks and further training and qualifications.

Leisure and Community Services managed the project for the first two years, by which time a management committee of local parents and professionals had been established and the project had been set up as a voluntary organisation. The management committee is currently chaired by a parent and the honorary officers are also parents.

In 1999, the Billesley area was chosen as one of the country's first 60 SureStart Trailblazer programmes, largely because of the existing work and services provided by the Chinnbrook Children and Parents' Project. Chinnbrook's history of working in partnership with parents, and providing services to meet their identified needs, was a good foundation on which to build a SureStart programme and it already met many of the SureStart criteria. The intention, over time, is to develop the capacity of the Chinnbrook Children and Parents' Project so that its management committee will be able to take responsibility for the management of the SureStart Billesley programme.

A visitor to the project is always warmly welcomed. It is often difficult to tell whether the person greeting you is a parent or a member of staff, as they all work together as a team. Whilst parents understand the boundaries between staff and parents, and respect these boundaries, they are completely at ease with staff and know that they will be listened to and that their views will be valued. Differences of opinion between staff and parents are not a threat, as negotiation is a regular feature of Chinnbrook.

I was associated with the project at a difficult time for them. The SureStart Billesley programme was just starting to take effect, and the staff of the project had been supporting the development of the SureStart programme in addition to their usual heavy workload. Parents and professionals on the management team were feeling out of their depth and under pressure to take on the management of the SureStart programme. The SureStart programme had a budget of £2.3 m over three years. The usual budget for Chinnbrook was around £70,000. Because the Chinnbrook project had always worked in partnership with parents and professionals in the area, finding solutions to problems together was not a new experience for them. They shared their thoughts openly, discussed the issues and decided jointly to take a step back from the situation, regain their confidence by refocusing on the Chinnbrook project and review the management of the SureStart programme at a later date. Parents on the management team felt listened to and understood. Even though they are volunteers, they stayed with the project through this difficult time and have emerged, as the staff have, stronger, maybe a little wiser and determined to ensure the project's continuing success.

WHAT IS THE FUTURE FOR PARENT PARTNERSHIP?

The future for services, like the two cited above, is to continue the process for, as has previously been stated, parent partnership is a process. Any partnership goes through its rough and its smooth times. All partnerships are dynamic, in the sense that they do not stay the same.

It is important not to become complacent. You may think that you have all the answers but will no doubt find that you have to reassess this when your team goes through a period of change or begins to work with a new group of parents.

You may have experienced what Marsh & Fisher (1992) referred to as the DATA effect, i.e. 'we **D**o **A**ll **T**his **A**lready'. They point out that:

> Workers *wanted* to base their work on what clients agreed should be done, they *believed* in the idea of participation . . . Given these genuine desires, their practice must, they considered, reflect them . . .

Marsh & Fisher found that often workers were not open to new ideas, because they felt they were already practising what they were being asked to do. However, they discovered that the methods of intervention, as experienced by users, did not match up to the way workers had described their practice methods.

The future for parent partnership is *you*. You have the power to make change. Even if the change is small, it will make a difference. Even if you cannot achieve major changes in your team, you can make changes in the way *you* work with parents. You can value and listen to them. You can include them in all decisions that relate to the provision of services to them. You can ensure that others in the team begin to see the value of parent partnership. I believe we all have a responsibility to do this. After all, it is a human right to be treated as an equal.

KEY POINTS

- Parent partnership means that the planning, development, delivery and monitoring of services are shared between the professionals/organisation providing services to parents and the parents who use the services.
- The combined effort of parents and professionals means that extra skills are available to both.
- Services that are designed and developed in partnership will be more relevant to service users' needs.
- Apathy is the greatest barrier to partnership working.
- The healthcare team can only move towards working in partnership with parents if there is a sincere willingness on the part of every member of the team to work in partnership.
- Working in partnership empowers both professionals and parents.

REFERENCES

Appleton P, Minchom P 1991 Models of parent partnership and child development centres. Child Care, Health and Development 17: 27–38

Cunningham C, Davis H 1985 Working with parents: frameworks for collaboration. Open University Press, Buckingham

Dale N 1996 Working with families of children with special needs: partnership and practice. Routledge, London

Marsh P, Fisher M 1992 Good intentions: developing partnership in social services. Joseph Rowntree Foundation, York

Mittler P, Mittler H 1983 Partnership with parents: an overview. In: Mittler P, McConachie H (eds) Parents, professionals and mentally handicapped people: approaches to partnership. Croom Helm, Beckenham, pp 10–11

Pugh G, De'Ath E 1989 Working towards partnership in the early years. National Children's Bureau, London

Wolfendale S 1983 Parental participation in children's development and education. Gordon and Breach Science Publishers, London

RESOURCES

KIDS, 6 Aztec Row, Berners Road, London N1 0PW
Tel: 020 7359 3635

Chinnbrook Children and Parents' Project, c/o 109 Trittiford Road, Billesley, Birmingham B13 0ET
Tel: 0121 443 4772

5 Antenatal education for parenting

Judith Ockenden

INTRODUCTION

The thing about having a baby is that thereafter you have it. (Quentin Crisp, in Saavedra 1992:8)

With small families and separation from relatives, many parents now have little or no experience of basic babycare skills. With universal medicalisation of perinatal care, they have learnt to rely on others and to wait to be told what to do. They now have to seek out support networks to fill the void left by the breakdown of close communities and extended families and to help them regain the skills and confidence they have lost.

A succession of childcare gurus has advised parents over the last century, from Dr Spock to Miriam Stoppard. Much of this advice is conflicting. Doctors, midwives, health visitors and well-meaning friends and relations are all eager to advise on practical aspects of care.

...advice has changed over time and has reflected not so much the needs of parents as the social and cultural norms of society and the influence of successive groups of professionals. (Pugh et al 1994)

Remarkably little work has been done on discovering what parents actually want (Nolan 1999) but there is now an increasing awareness of the need to consider the social and emotional implications of having a baby (Ockenden 2000 and references therein) and to respond to the individual needs of parents. This chapter describes a variety of educational approaches to help expectant parents think about life after the birth of their baby. For ideas specific to the needs of fathers-to-be, see Chapter 6.

WHAT DO PARENTS WANT?

Until recently, received wisdom was that it is very difficult to interest pregnant women in postnatal issues because they are so focused on the birth. And (the logic follows), if they are not interested, they are not motivated and therefore will not learn (Daines et al 1993, Rogers 1989).

Conversely, whenever parents have been asked, after the birth, about their antenatal classes, they say that they were deficient in practical and emotional aspects of postnatal life (Nolan 1997). In a recent survey of NCT services (Holmes & Newburn 1999), 67% of parents said classes were very helpful for labour but only 21% said the same for the early postnatal period – looking after their baby, what to expect and coping with physical changes and emotions. This evidence backs up what any antenatal teacher who evaluates classes will tell you (with a sigh): retrospective evaluation *always* asks for more on postnatal issues.

But what about prospective research? Is this antenatal/postnatal divide a true paradox or is it based on false assumptions, failure to ask the right questions and lack of skill in interesting parents in issues we know will be relevant to them after the birth?

A recent antenatal study (Nolan 1999) shows that both parents are keen to acquire confidence and skills to (a) use the healthcare system effectively, (b) care for their babies and (c) make decisions about their families' health and care. Men, in particular, are keen to learn about postnatal issues and it is important to consider them equally, acknowledging that in many respects they have a different perspective on becoming a parent (see Chapter 6).

Later I will describe practical ways of stimulating thoughts about parenting but first I would like to consider why parents need preparation at this time.

THE TRANSITION TO PARENTHOOD

Traditionally, transition to parenthood has been defined as beginning with the confirmation of pregnancy and ending a few months after the birth. There is a good case, however, for extending this period. Polomeno (2000) describes nine phases in the transition, beginning with the decision to have a baby and ending when the child is two years old. This echoes the assertion of Corwin (1999) that the couple should already be regarded as parents antenatally; there are already three people in the relationship. It is also a similar time period to that of adjustment to other major life transitions.

> *While a baby is gestating, so is motherhood. When a baby is born, so are its mother and father 'born'.* (England & Horowitz 1998:256)

During pregnancy the mother becomes accustomed to the physical dependence of her developing baby and the father can see the growing evidence of this. Both parents begin to experience changes in perspectives on life, changes in their sex life and changes in their emotional and social interactions. Postnatally the child is dependent on all levels, psychological, emotional and physical, and the latter needs are no longer dealt with automatically (Corwin 1999).

Corwin (1998) writes that babies, when awake, are typically contented and have 'no needs' for only about 15 minutes of every hour. She goes on to say that having to meet the needs of the infant for 45 minutes of many hours sometimes comes as a surprise to first-time parents. I would say it often comes as a nasty shock. And I would agree that it can and often does give rise to parental emotional distress.

> *. . . they will probably feel like the first three months are interminable . . .* (Corwin 1999:26)

Babies do sleep a lot in the first few weeks and months of life but their sleeping pattern is usually not predictable and doesn't fit in with that of their parents. Sleep deprivation can have profound effects on both the mental health of the parents and on their relationship (Larkin & Butler 2000). The realities of new parenthood are hugely different from advertising images. One of the mothers under study in Belsky & Kelly (1994) compared the difference in the anticipated impact of the baby on the family and the reality to 'watching a tornado on TV and having one actually blow the roof off your house'.

Underdown (1998) suggests that parents have a 'fantasy of fusion' during pregnancy, which can lead to an unreal expectation of closeness after the baby is born. Belsky & Kelly (1994) consider that the mother's priority then becomes the baby while the father redoubles his old priorities, such as work. These researchers studied 250 couples from the third trimester of pregnancy until the child's third birthday. The condition of the marriage at the end of the study compared to at the beginning was assessed and put into one of four categories: 12% were severe decliners; 39% were moderate decliners; 30% had no change; 19% were improvers.

In the absence of understanding and validation . . . there can be stagnation and gradual deterioration, a diminution of shared experiences and a decline in appreciation and affection. (Polomeno 2000:34)

England & Horowitz (1998:262) describe the areas of most conflict in a marriage after the birth of a baby:

- division of labour
- money
- work
- relationships/communication
- social life.

These factors correspond closely to the 'six domains in the transition to parenthood' cited by Underdown (1998). To adapt successfully to parenthood, couples must:

- work together as a team
- sort out roles
- cope with stress and avoid stressing the partner
- argue constructively
- acknowledge that their relationship has changed
- communicate and sustain common interests.

. . . if a couple does not successfully adapt to each stage of conjugal life, unresolved emotional issues carry into the next stage . . . [which] could eventually result in emotional withdrawal . . . (Polomeno 2000:34–35)

Perhaps couples in the first of Polomeno's (2000) nine phases of transition – Decision to become pregnant – should follow the suggestion of Leonhardt-Lupa (1995:133), to renew their marriage vows.

How can educators help in the metamorphosis from couple to family?

EASING THE TRANSITION

It has been shown that even a small amount of intervention in the first year can have a significant impact on improving the experience of parenting and reducing separation (Underdown 1998). Polomeno (2000) has devised a detailed plan for the perinatal period: in this chapter it is her 'primary prevention' that we are concerned with – modifying external conditions and/or offering coping strategies to avoid problems before they start. Antenatal classes are often the only opportunity to do this.

Dawn Robinson-Walsh (1996) quotes her partner:

Having children gives you something to work for as a couple, to pull in the same direction for. They add extra meaning to life, a new dimension.

She adds: 'How right this is, but how hard it can be'.

We need to prepare parents for 'how hard it can be'. Polomeno (2000) describes 'sensitising' parents, giving 'anticipatory guidance' and 'skill building'. Nolan (1998) discusses 'the anticipatory work of worrying'. They need to know that conjugal strain is normal at critical times, that there will inevitably be a period of disorganisation and reorganisation. There will be losses, both temporary and permanent, but there will also be tremendous gains. Life will be good in a different way.

O'Driscoll (1998) suggests that guilt and resentment are the two biggest destroyers of relationships. To avoid guilt, couples need to:

- anticipate their roles after the birth and either accept them or work out other ways of doing things
- have realistic expectations of what life will be like and also of themselves
- understand that it is not their fault if their baby's behaviour differs from the 'norm' (Page 2000:368)
- be able to speak assertively to their partner about their needs and to make time to nurture their relationship
- know that it may take some time to reestablish their full sex life and that that will be facilitated if they feel mentally and physically well.

You, the educator, must find a variety of ways to inculcate these messages.

LISTENING AND INFORMING

I tend to agree with a statement attributed to Erica Jong (in Saavedra 1992): 'Advice is what we ask for when we already know the answer but wish we didn't'.

If, for example, a woman asks you, 'How can I make my baby sleep?', she almost certainly knows that there is no safe way to *make* him or her do so. She is really asking for several things:

- someone to listen to her problem
- someone to empathise with her problem
- information about what is 'normal' regarding babies' sleeping patterns
- reassurance that her baby's behaviour and her reaction to it are 'normal'
- coping strategies to soothe her baby
- coping strategies to avoid getting distressed and get some rest
- possible strategies she can use to encourage her baby to develop sleeping patterns which help her to get more sleep.

In this situation, simply saying, for example, 'leave her to cry' is useless if she is totally opposed to doing so or if her baby is the kind who makes herself sick if she is left. Similarly, saying 'sleep with him in your bed' won't suit someone who doesn't get a wink of sleep if her baby is in her bed or simply doesn't want him there. Information about a variety of ideas will allow her to select a way forward suited to her (and her partner). As Judith Schott (1994) said:

> How would it be if, instead of giving advice, which is often conflicting and sometimes inappropriate, we listened to the woman and encouraged her to talk about what is important to her? . . . The woman may spontaneously find her own solutions, but, if not, by understanding her situation more fully, we are in a better position to offer the information (not advice) she needs in order to make her own decisions.

So, education is not the same thing as advice giving. Neither is information the same thing as advice. Information is extremely important, because:

> Lack of information has direct effects on limiting informed choice, increasing dependence and engendering passivity, with implications for control, fear and a lack of cognitive preparation. (Sherr 1995:135)

Giving information is the role of the educator; deciding how to use it is up to the parent. Telling people what to do merely reinforces the power/subservience relationship. It does nothing to enable parents to develop self-confidence or acquire skills appropriate to their situation.

If an educator finds a parent holds mistaken or even worrying attitudes:

> We need to recognise and respond to the fear that often lies behind extreme decisions or entrenched attitudes. Listening without judgement, and showing respect, empathy and acceptance can, in itself be healing and allow for change . . . (Smith 1998:3)

May (2000) has described the results of following the ethos described, for example, in Nolan (1998): asking parents what they want; working in small groups; problem solving; informal discussions; building a support network. She writes:

> We have learnt . . . that what we as educators can tell parents is marginal. What we can do is support couples in developing confidence and self-esteem as they approach the challenges of becoming new parents. (May 2000:45)

SETTING THE AGENDA

It is important to find out what, in particular, parents want to know, to increase their motivation to learn (Priest & Schott 1991). This can be done by consulting and negotiating within a framework in which they can express their needs (Daines et al 1993:28–31; Nolan 1998:122).

Simply asking parents at the beginning of a course what they want to cover may leave them floundering. They may assume that the classes are only about preparing for the birth and so request only birth-related issues. Thus, they need to know the aims of the course – the underlying philosophy and hopes of the educator.

ACTIVITY 5.1

AGENDA SETTING

Show the class a large cross-sectional picture of a non-pregnant woman (showing the uterus and other organs). Ask if anyone can remember being like this?

Say that the women have been going through a time of tremendous change. Produce another chart of a woman at a stage of pregnancy roughly equivalent to that of the parents in the class.

Say that the baby too has been undergoing remarkable development. A new family has been created. The couples may have already noticed that their relationship had subtly changed.

Now show the chart of a pregnant woman at term. In just a few weeks, the birth will be happening and 24 hours later the parents in the class will have . . .

Produce a realistic baby doll. Pause for thought.

Then produce another, larger doll, pointing out that in just a few months they will be parents of a person more like 'this'.

Comment that, in the space of 18 months, they will have gone from 'this' (the non-pregnant chart) to having a small person in their life (the larger doll).

The aim of these classes is to enable you to look back in a year's time feeling that your experience of all these changes has been as satisfying and rewarding as possible.

Now, on flipchart paper, ask the parents to write words or phrases, or draw pictures, about what aspects of this time of change they feel will be challenging, interesting or worrying; in other words, what would they like to cover in the classes?

The results of this exercise used at a recent class were as follows.

- Drinking
- Factual information
- Birth plan
- Pain
- Pain control in labour
- Epidurals
- Water births
- The most helpful things blokes can do in labour
- Losing control
- Will I lose the weight?
- What is normal?
- Sleep
- Sleep pattern
- Sleep deprivation
- Who to ask
- Feeding
- Screaming
- Smelly nappies
- What equipment is needed?
- Childcare
- Time (lack of)
- Not forgetting each other and how to enjoy life
- How much time to have off work
- Going back to work
- Going out
- Grandparents
- Parents/Christening/Pressure!

Six couples attending a recent course I ran (Activity 5.1) identified seven issues specifically related to birth, four general points and 16 postnatal 'wants'. An alternative exercise is shown in Activity 5.2.

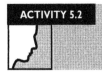

ACTIVITY 5.2 Write a key word (baby?) in the middle of the flipchart. By word association, demonstrating chains of thought, the class members reveal the questions and worries that are at the forefront of their minds.

The postnatal issues identified by the six couples who completed Activity 5.1 enabled me to establish aims and learning outcomes relating to parenting for their antenatal course.

Aims

- To promote the mental and physical well-being of the parents.
- To enable the parents to achieve a satisfying lifestyle and fulfilling relationships.
- To boost the parents' confidence in their ability to look after themselves and their baby.
- To enable the parents to have realistic expectations about their baby's feeding and sleeping behaviour and about physical recovery from birth and mental adjustment to parenthood.

Learning outcomes

By the end of this course, the parents would:

- be able to demonstrate practical babycare skills
- have coping strategies for catching up on rest and sleep, making time for essential jobs and relationships, and for relieving stress
- be able to demonstrate assertiveness skills to reject unrealistic role models and politely decline unwelcome advice
- have peer group and family networks in place and know where they could access professional and voluntary group support, and how to ask for it.

ACTIVITIES FOR PARENTHOOD PREPARATION

There follows a series of activities to address the aims and learning outcomes listed above.

Transition to parenthood

To set parents off thinking about the transition to parenthood, try Activity 5.3.

ACTIVITY 5.3

POSTNATAL TIME LINE

In small groups (four if enough people), ask what is happening – physically, emotionally, medically, practically – to Mum, Dad and Baby:

- 1–3 hours after birth
- 2–3 days after birth
- 3 weeks after birth
- 3 months after birth.

Ask them to think about post-vaginal and post-caesarean births. They can write down their thoughts on a large piece of flipchart paper and then share them with the larger group.

Sleep

The topic of sleep came up three times during the agenda-setting exercise, reflecting its importance both in anticipation and in reality.

> *People who say they sleep like a baby usually don't have one.* (Leo J Burke, in Saavedra 1992:35)

Sleeping patterns are closely linked with feeding behaviour in young babies (Leach 1999) and can be illustrated by either of the next two activities (5.4 and 5.5).

ACTIVITY 5.4

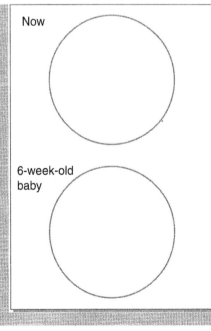

Now

6-week-old baby

24-HOUR CLOCK

Give each parent an A4 sheet.

Ask them to choose a day over the past week and fill in the 24-hour clock of their life activities – working, sleeping, cleaning, relaxing, etc.

Then, remind them that a baby of 6 weeks might sleep, on average, 10–12 hours in 24, feed (say) eight times and that each feed might occupy up to an hour. Ask them to draw a new clock for a day when the baby is 6 weeks old.

Discuss the results.

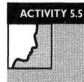

ACTIVITY 5.5

FEEDING STARS

Make five coloured cards, about 40 cm long and 15 cm wide. Number them 1 to 5 to represent 5 days in the life of a baby, say during the second week of life. Stick gold stars randomly along the length of the card, each one representing a feed.

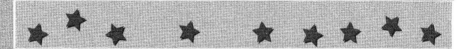

Remember that babies can feed between six and 14 times during a 24-hour period. Use the visual display to trigger a discussion about feeding and sleeping.

This exercise could be adapted to any time period you wanted to highlight or could be used to represent five different babies instead of five days for one baby.

Prioritising

First-time parents may be daunted by the issues raised by these activities. Either in the same class or following up in the next one, begin to introduce ways of coping with the new challenges. Activities 5.6 and 5.7 could be done by two small groups at the same time.

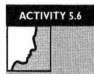

ACTIVITY 5.6

WHO DOES WHAT?

On four A4 header sheets, write in large lettering:

1. man usually does this
2. woman usually does this
3. we usually do this together
4. someone else usually does this.

On small cards (about 4 cm square), write down as many household tasks as you can think of – before a baby is born. Include paying bills, gardening and maintenance, as well as washing, ironing and cleaning. Ask the couples to arrange the postcards on to the relevant A4 sheets. A consensus view is OK if several couples are doing the task together, or they might choose one couple in the group to represent them.

Now introduce some different-coloured squares with baby-oriented tasks on them, including soothing and comforting as well as feeding and changing. Ask them to imagine the baby is 6 weeks old. They must rearrange the existing cards and add the new baby cards to show how they envisage things with a 6-week-old baby.

Ask:

- what, if anything, strikes you about the arrangement of the cards?
- what did you agree/disagree about?
- do you foresee any problems with these arrangements?
- if you had a fifth sheet, 'Don't do for the time being', would you put anything on it?

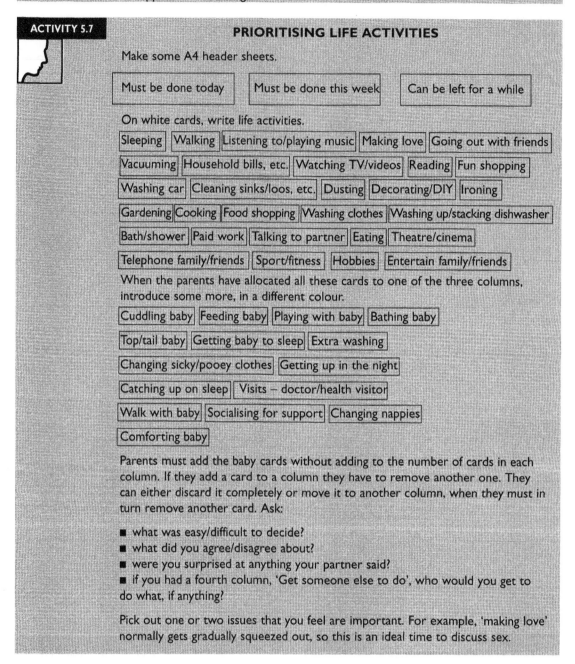

ACTIVITY 5.7

PRIORITISING LIFE ACTIVITIES

Make some A4 header sheets.

| Must be done today | Must be done this week | Can be left for a while |

On white cards, write life activities.

Sleeping | Walking | Listening to/playing music | Making love | Going out with friends

Vacuuming | Household bills, etc. | Watching TV/videos | Reading | Fun shopping

Washing car | Cleaning sinks/loos, etc. | Dusting | Decorating/DIY | Ironing

Gardening | Cooking | Food shopping | Washing clothes | Washing up/stacking dishwasher

Bath/shower | Paid work | Talking to partner | Eating | Theatre/cinema

Telephone family/friends | Sport/fitness | Hobbies | Entertain family/friends

When the parents have allocated all these cards to one of the three columns, introduce some more, in a different colour.

Cuddling baby | Feeding baby | Playing with baby | Bathing baby

Top/tail baby | Getting baby to sleep | Extra washing

Changing sicky/pooey clothes | Getting up in the night

Catching up on sleep | Visits – doctor/health visitor

Walk with baby | Socialising for support | Changing nappies

Comforting baby

Parents must add the baby cards without adding to the number of cards in each column. If they add a card to a column they have to remove another one. They can either discard it completely or move it to another column, when they must in turn remove another card. Ask:

■ what was easy/difficult to decide?
■ what did you agree/disagree about?
■ were you surprised at anything your partner said?
■ if you had a fourth column, 'Get someone else to do', who would you get to do what, if anything?

Pick out one or two issues that you feel are important. For example, 'making love' normally gets gradually squeezed out, so this is an ideal time to discuss sex.

Sleep deprivation

It is important that parents know the problems of sleep deprivation (Larkin & Butler 2000). Activity 5.8 could be used to introduce these ideas.

ACTIVITY 5.8   Ask if anyone has had experience of sleep deprivation, perhaps in their job. What effects does it have? How do you cope?

So, given that early parenting is likely to result in sleep deprivation, how can its effects be minimised? Encourage parents to put rest first with Activity 5.9.

ACTIVITY 5.9

REST AND SLEEP

Scatter some quotation cards* and ask each person to take one. The same quotation can be repeated several times if necessary.

Rest is not idleness (Sir James Lubbock).

There was no need to do any housework at all. After the first four years, the dirt doesn't get any worse (Quentin Crisp).

Keeping house is like threading beads on a string with no knot at the end (Anon.).

Dull people have tidy homes (Anon.).

Hatred of domestic work is a natural and admirable result of civilisation (Rebecca West).

One of the advantages of being disorderly is that one is constantly making exciting discoveries (A A Milne).

The time to relax is when you don't have time for it (Sydney J Harris).

Ask someone to read out each card and discuss it. Do they agree? Do they agree with their partner? Even if they are normally very tidy, could they accept a lowering of standards for a while? Could they ask someone to help them, even temporarily? If they agree with the sentiments of the card, can they uphold this philosophy against perceived expectations of friends, relatives and the 'I must' voices inside them?

Invite them to take the card home and display it in a prominent place.
*These were taken from Saavedra (1992) and *The Oxford Dictionary of Phrase, Saying and Quotation* (1997).

Relaxation

Follow this activity with a relaxation exercise (Activity 5.10).

ACTIVITY 5.10

PUTTING REST FIRST

Pick up a realistic baby doll and hold it tenderly as you would a real baby. Ask everyone to sit comfortably and imagine being in the situation you are going to describe. Invite them to close their eyes.

Your partner has gone out for the afternoon for a well-deserved break with friends. You are looking after your 3-week-old baby. If you are a father and your baby is being breastfed, you have a supply of expressed milk to feed to your baby in a bottle. You didn't get much sleep last night, so you are hoping to have a nap, then tidy up the house and prepare a simple meal, perhaps with a glass of good wine.

At first your baby is quietly alert. You hold her facing you and talk to her and she makes funny faces and blows bubbles. She's absolutely delightful and you're looking forward to the hours ahead. After a while, you both get a bit bored with this, so you decide to put her in her bouncy chair while you tidy up around her.

Unfortunately, every time you put her down she begins to cry. So you go in search of the baby sling. She usually falls asleep in that when you go for a walk. As you are putting her in the sling, there is a tremendous reverberation and you realise she has just filled her nappy. On changing her you see that she has leaked onto her clothes, so you wash and change her too.

She is now much happier and allows you to spend 5 minutes tidying the kitchen while watching you from her bouncy chair. She then begins to get restless, doing the familiar sideways turn of her head and movement of her mouth which tells you she is hungry. Quickly finishing the washing up, you take her to a comfortable chair in the sitting room, arrange cushions, a drink, the telephone and the TV remote around you. You slide off your shoes. You begin to feed the baby.

After feeding, burping and feeding again, your baby is now fast asleep on your chest. Your 'I must' voice tells you to tidy up, but you are very tired and know it will be difficult to cope with the baby and meal preparation later if you don't get a little sleep. You look at the mantelpiece and see the card you got from the antenatal class.

'Rest is not idleness'

You close your eyes and let your shoulders drop and then your jaw. You stretch your legs and let your thighs sink into the chair. You are aware of breathing, slowly and deeply into your abdomen, and of the long outward breath, taking your tension with it. You can hear your baby breathing rhythmically and smell the lovely scent of her head.

For a while your body and mind have the opportunity to replenish their reserves. And the closeness to your sleeping baby fills you with feelings of love and protectiveness.

After some time, you rouse yourself. The baby is still asleep so you gently put her onto the warm patch on the chair where you have been sitting and cover her with a shawl. You go into the kitchen to prepare the meal.

Debriefing

Role models are very important in parenting (Raphael-Leff 1991:332). If the mother and father have had different experiences they may not agree on how to look after their child. Guilt can be engendered too if they feel they cannot live up to their inner image of a perfect parent – an image created from many positive and negative experiences and observations (Giles 1997). Debriefing may help with this and give the couples time to discuss any differences before the birth. Debriefing has to be done with great care in case individuals' experiences have been painful (Activity 5.11).

ACTIVITY 5.11

DEBRIEFING (from Smith, 1998)

In pairs, participants ask each other: 'What would you want for your child as he or she grows up?' The educator explains that group members may describe things they had or didn't have themselves as a child and stresses that they only have to reveal what they want to in this situation.

Babyproofing the couple's relationship

Earlier in this chapter, we discussed how many relationships deteriorate after the birth of a baby. The activities promoting realistic expectations and coping strategies will begin to prepare couples (see also Activity 5.12), but what

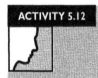

ACTIVITY 5.12

POSTPARTUM ADJUSTMENT PLAN
(adapted from England & Horowitz, 1998:263)

There are five things that tend to divide couples: division of labour, money, work, relationship problems and social life.

1. Think of your own relationship and, without consulting your partner, write down which of these issues – or any others – could be potential problems for you. You will not have to share these things with other couples in the class.
2. With your partner, share your concerns. Listen without interrupting while your partner talks. Try to accept your partner's view even if it surprises or upsets you.
3. Together, think of and write down any possible solutions to the potential problems, even if some seem unrealistic.
4. From this list, choose one or two strategies that seem most likely to ease each problem. Highlight them in some way.
5. Display this list on your noticeboard at home or next to your favourite saying on your mantelpiece. And USE IT.

This could be an exercise that you encourage couples to do at home, particularly if you are running single-sex classes.

other exercises might help in babyproofing a marriage? This expression is not to suggest that parents should make themselves impervious to their child's needs, but that they allow themselves to enjoy parenthood without damage, just as waterproof clothing allows one to enjoy going out without getting wet and cold.

What is normal?

To address the 'What is normal?' question, try using a questionnaire (Figure 5.1).

It is not necessary to 'mark' the answers. Initiate a discussion by asking class members if anything surprised them.

| FIGURE 5.1 | *Postnatal quiz* |

Please circle the figure you think is correct

1. What percentage of babies still wake regularly at 1 year?

    (25%)   50%   75%

2. What percentage of couples say their marriage is improved after the birth of a baby?

    (20%)   50%   75%

3. On average, how much less frequently do couples make love in the first year after a baby is born?

    10%   (40%)   70%

4. What percentage of mothers think that their partner does not pull his weight at home?

    25%   50%   (75%)

5. How many women suffer from:

    (a) puerperal psychosis?

    (0.2%)   2%   10%

    (b) clinical postnatal depression?

    1%   (10%)   20%

    (c) baby blues?

    20%   50%   (70%)

A similar quiz could be devised about babies' behaviour. Another way to help normalise postnatal problems is to promote the formation of a self-help group among the class attenders. Encourage them to arrange a meeting in the week following the end of the classes and a reunion when all their babies are born.

Comparing common experiences provides ongoing support. (Polomeno 2000:37)

Changing self-image

Concern about losing the weight she has gained during pregnancy reflects a woman's worry about her changing body image. Use 'trigger' pictures to stimulate ideas and debate (Activity 5.13).

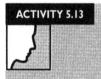

ACTIVITY 5.13

Use a variety of different images of women – with partner, with children, at work, at play and leisure. Invite each class member to choose a picture and say why he or she has chosen this one. Encourage a discussion. How are they going to enjoy themselves with the baby, as a couple and as individuals? How are they going to

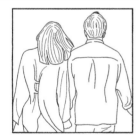 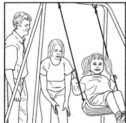 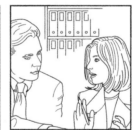 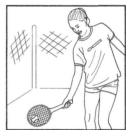

make sure they get enough good food and exercise? Why do women tend to put on weight when they have a baby? Provide a list of exercise classes in your area for mothers with babies – yoga, aquanatal, etc.

Remind class members that it's normal for a woman to be 'out of shape' when she's had a baby. It helps to keep a sense of humour about it.

Don't kid yourself. Those women [on Jane Fonda's exercise tape] have never had babies. Their children were all borne by professional stunt women. (Dave Barry, in Saavedra 1992: 159)

Assertiveness

To have time to themselves, individually and as a couple, parents need to be able to ask for help. They can ask each other for time on their own (Activity 5.14). They may be able to ask friends and relations to babysit.

> *People sometimes think of immaturity as being too dependent. Another kind of immaturity is not being able to ask for help.* (England & Horowitz 1998:257)

ACTIVITY 5.14

ASSERTIVENESS

When the baby is 3 weeks old, a breastfeeding mother wants to go out shopping on her own. She would like her partner to look after the baby for a couple of hours.

Scenario 1

Woman	I'm going shopping on my own this afternoon. I'm absolutely sick of having no time to myself.
Man	But what if the baby gets hungry?
Woman	I knew you'd say that. You don't want me to go do you?
Man	Oh, here we go. I suppose you're going to sulk now?
Woman (shouting)	No, I'm taking the baby out shopping with me as usual!
Man (shouting)	Fine, you do that!

Scenario 2

Woman	I'm really feeling in need of a couple of hours to myself.
Man	I'm not surprised. What do you want to do?
Woman	Well, I've been wearing these elasticated trousers so much over the last few months, I'd love to go and choose something new to wear.
Man	Could you go just after you've fed the baby?
Woman	Yes, and there's a couple of ounces of expressed milk in the freezer which I could get out just in case.
Man	Fine, I'll probably take her out for a walk so she'll sleep most of the time anyway.
Woman	Great. I'll bring a take-away back!

Discuss the differences between the two scenarios, i.e. the difference between aggressive demands and assertive negotiation. Hopefully, this will raise a smile but the message will be a strong one.

The scenarios could be adapted for conversations with grandparents, perhaps. And instead of providing a scenario, you could ask the class members to devise their own.

Support

It is important to help women and men think carefully about where their support will come from after their baby has been born. Try Activity 5.15.

ACTIVITY 5.15

SUPPORT NETWORK

Give each couple a sheet.

Who do you know who . . .

■ accepts you as you are?
■ is reliable in a crisis?
■ knows the pleasures and pitfalls of parenthood?
■ is willing to help out without making you feel you owe them something?
■ is a good listener?
■ puts things into perspective?
■ has time to help?
■ can be paid to help?
■ can put you in touch with useful people/organisations?

Ask the whole group whether they managed to find somebody for each category. (You, the educator, are in the last category.) There may be those who have few friends or relatives in the area, perhaps because they have recently moved. Talk about local support groups and exercise opportunities for new mothers where they can meet new friends. Again, encourage the group to continue to meet after the classes.

Postnatal depression

Parents-to-be are very aware of the high prevalence of postnatal depression, although they might not know that men can suffer from it as well as women. Helping them understand more about depression and enabling them to recognise it is a very useful aspect of antenatal classes (Activity 5.16).

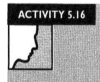

ACTIVITY 5.16

POSTNATAL DEPRESSION (adapted from Nolan 1998:135)

Set out three large cards.

| Normal | ? | Depressed |

Prepare some small cards with symptoms that might or might not be signs of clinical depression, for example:

Cries all day a few days after the baby is born; Can't stop eating; Loses appetite; Won't let baby out of her sight; Can't bear the baby crying; Always tired; Thinks about suicide; Thinks about harming her baby; Avoids other people; Insomnia; Wants to sleep all the time; Can't concentrate; Losing weight; Always complaining of aches and pains; Suffers from many headaches; Irritable; Feels guilty; Feels incompetent; Worries about small things; Can't be bothered

Give a few cards to each parent, ask them to read each card out and choose a heading for it to go under. Much discussion should follow about what is/isn't normal. The educator can draw out the following key issues.

- It is usually a combination of symptoms rather than a single one that is worrying.
- Different people show different symptoms.
- The difference between 'baby blues', depression and puerperal psychosis.
- The importance of the woman or her partner seeking help from health professionals if they think they may be clinically depressed.
- Combined drug therapy and counselling is effective and non-addictive.
- Dads can get depressed too!

Returning to paid work

While more and more women go back to work after having a baby, society remains ambivalent about whether it would prefer its mothers in the workforce or at home with their children. Antenatal classes provide an opportunity for parents to think through the pressures that will be acting upon them and how they might cope (Activity 5.17).

ACTIVITY 5.17   **RETURNING TO PAID WORK**

Divide the class into four groups, if there are enough people. Provide each with a picture and a large piece of paper.

Each group has 5 minutes to write down the thoughts evoked by their picture.

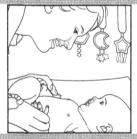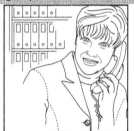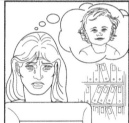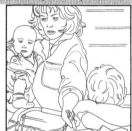

A key question might help. For example, 'What is the image of a full-time mother in our society? What are the advantages/disadvantages of returning to work? If you want to go back to work, how long would you like to take off if you had the choice?'

They then pass their picture and paper on to the next group. This time they have 4 minutes. The pictures are 'snowballed' for another 3, then 2 minutes.

The thoughts are then pooled into the whole group and a discussion follows about the pros and cons of working/staying at home/combining the two.

This can be followed up with a discussion about childcare, giving information about where to find out about local nurseries and childminders.

Statements on cards about people's different perceptions of full-time motherhood and returning to paid work could also be used for this activity, e.g.:

It seems to me that life is all about choice and sacrifice. (Knox 1997)
Nothing has a stronger influence psychologically on their environment, and especially on their children, than the unlived life of the parents. (CG Jung, in Saavedra 1992:91)

Babycare skills

Towards the end of the antenatal course, when the birth is imminent, parents may begin to wonder just what they are going to do with their baby when they take him home and may be very receptive to practising babycare skills (Activities 5.18 and 5.19).

ACTIVITY 5.18

BATHING AT BEDTIME

Gather together some props: a realistic baby doll (soft-bodied ones handle more like real babies), a baby bath or washing-up bowl (no water if it's a soft-bodied doll!), changing mat, nappies, cotton wool, wipes, lotions and potions, towel, clothes, and a small cot or Moses basket with bedding.

Ask one parent (possibly a Dad because it might be uncomfortable for the Mums) to volunteer to bath the baby and put it to bed. Ask him to hold the doll (which has a nappy on and is wrapped in a shawl). He must now treat the doll as if it were a real baby.

Ask the other group members, 'What does he do first?', 'What does he do next?'. Make sure key issues are addressed. Has he tested the water temperature and how should he do that? Does he need to use that cream? Which way round does the nappy go? Is he going to use the disposable or washable kind? How does he put the baby down to sleep?

Many babycare issues will be raised by this exercise (e.g. What equipment do you need? Where will your baby sleep?) as well as its being a demonstration of practical skills.

Changing nappies

Provide a selection of baby dolls with 'dirty' nappies. Smear Marmite or peanut butter on the nappies to represent meconium and a breastfed baby's nappy. This causes great hilarity and is good for the class bonding!

Discuss whether group members are considering using disposable or washable nappies. Invite someone from the Real Nappy Network to demonstrate the range that is now available or get some samples or pictures to show.

Issues such as nappy rash and how often you need to change a baby are likely to be raised.

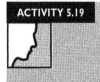

ACTIVITY 5.19

SOOTHING A CRYING BABY

Invest in a realistic baby doll that cries or use a non-crying doll with a tape of a crying baby. As the doll is passed around the room, each class member has to describe or demonstrate a different way of trying to stop the crying. The noise very quickly becomes stressful and the relief is immense when you finally turn it off!

Help group members understand the following.

■ That it is normal sometimes to feel very angry with your baby if she won't stop crying and even to feel you want to hurt the child. If you feel like that, put the baby down for a while and go out of the room until you compose yourself. If possible, ask your partner or a neighbour to give you a break. Try deep breathing and muscle-relaxing exercises. Make a cup of tea, put on some soothing music and start all over again. (This could be a good time to do the 'Putting rest first' relaxation described earlier.)

■ Signs that the baby might be unwell. Reassure them that GPs would rather you contact them if you are worried, even if it turns out to be a false alarm.

Taking the baby out is often suggested as a way of getting him to sleep. Use the opportunity to discuss slings, prams and car seats.

Parents learn well from their peers, so consider inviting some parents with a new baby of about 6 weeks to visit the class (Activity 5.20). (Any older than 6 weeks and the prospective parents might not identify with the baby.)

ACTIVITY 5.20

VISIT BY NEW PARENTS

Choose parents who will be honest about their experiences without making the class anxious and who will be comfortable being watched and questioned. Talk to them beforehand about why you have invited them and what sort of questions might be raised. Ask whether they are happy for others to hold their baby and whether the mother would be prepared to feed the baby in front of the group. Suggest a time when they might come and go.

Prime the class members with relevant questions, but invite them to use their own questions as well.

1. What is a typical day/night like with the baby?
2. How do you feel about the birth now?
3. What was your experience of hospital like?
4. Was it easy to breastfeed?
5. Do you manage to find time for yourselves?
6. What's the nicest thing about being a parent?
7. What's the worst thing about being a parent?
8. What do you wish you had known before labour/having a baby?
9. What pieces of baby equipment have you found most useful?

Don't rush to get the parents to leave, but ensure there is time for the group to debrief the meeting afterwards. Discuss any issues raised.

Infant feeding

To hone in on questions and worries about feeding, trigger pictures could be used again or the class members asked what experiences, if any, they have of friends or relatives feeding babies. Cultural and social influences are particularly strong regarding this subject.

Biological models of breastfeeding that do not give attention to individual experiences or to shared beliefs about the body mean that breastfeeding is often far more significant than professional wisdom allows. (Hames 1997:6)

If you have not been trained specifically in breastfeeding education, consider asking someone who has to lead this session. The subject of feeding babies is too big to cover in detail here, but a comprehensive list of possible topics to include in a breastfeeding class is given in Priest & Schott (1991:32) and excellent pointers for teaching can be found in Page (2000:369–383). Breast and bottle can be covered alongside each other in a way that emphasises the benefits of breast without stigmatising the bottle (Activity 5.21).

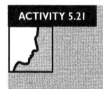

ACTIVITY 5.21

FEEDING (adapted from Nolan, 1998:76)

Using realistic, soft-bodied baby dolls, ask class members to demonstrate how they think you would hold a baby for (a) breastfeeding and (b) bottlefeeding. Elicit that closeness, skin contact and communication with the baby are possible however the baby is being fed. In both cases, mother needs to be comfortable so she can use feeding as an opportunity for rest and to enjoy her baby. Emphasise the 'chest-to-chest, nose-to-nipple' position essential for breastfeeding. Use good pictures to show correct and incorrect positioning and latch.

Discuss the constituents of breast and formula milk. Breastmilk is tailor made to babies' requirements. Formula manufacturers refine their product all the time, but formula milk cannot change throughout the feed as breastmilk does, nor as the baby grows. A breastfed baby gets a drink at the beginning of every feed to quench her thirst but a formula-fed baby will need some bottles of cool, boiled water once or twice a day to ensure he does not get thirsty.

As formula milk is a combination of chemicals, it is important to follow carefully the make-up instructions. Breastmilk is always the correct composition, readily available and sterile. Discuss sterilisation of equipment for bottlefeeding and storage of expressed breastmilk and formula.

Although bottlefeeding allows fathers and others to feed the baby, expressed breastmilk can also be given by someone other than the mother, using a sterile spoon or feeding cup. Discuss methods of initiating a breastfed baby into using a bottle and when to wean babies (breast or bottlefed) onto solids.

Enjoying parenting

One of the prospective fathers in the group who set the agenda referred to earlier in this chapter, complained that he was sick of people telling him about the 'bad stuff', and he wanted to hear some of the positive things about being a parent. Good point! (See Activity 5.22.)

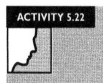

ACTIVITY 5.22

100 GOOD THINGS ABOUT BEING A PARENT

I recently downloaded a list with this title from an email group. It's too long to include here, but here are some examples:

■ rediscovering the sea the first time you show your toddler how to paddle
■ knowing you will pass on all your genes for wit, charm, beauty and modesty to your baby

- understanding just what your Mum and Dad did for you all those years ago to
- developing a new family language as your toddler talks about 'scissoring' the lawn or asks for drinks of 'duce'.

Compile your own list (ask around for ideas) and display it for parents.

One way of helping parents look forward to parenting is to focus on how they can encourage their baby's development (Activity 5.23).

ACTIVITY 5.23	**INFANT STIMULATION** (adapted from Nolan, 1998:155)	
Touch	Skin-to-skin contact and cuddling make babies grow and develop faster. Demonstrate baby massage or ask someone to come in to the class to do so. Perhaps one of the class members knows how to do this.
Hearing	Babies recognise their parents' voices from an early age – and even tunes which you played a lot while they were in the womb (Eastenders/The Archers!). They like rhythmical music. Ask the class members to relearn a nursery rhyme or lullaby and bring it to the next class. (They don't have to sing it.) Discuss how people talk to babies and why they use a certain pitch and intonation.
Sight	Babies like strong, contrasting colours for about the first 6 months. They also like to look at faces, particularly those of their parents. Ask parents to make a black-and-white mobile for their baby to look at.
Smell	Babies like sweet smells such as breastmilk or fruit. They also like your smell. Ask class members how they could use this fact to help soothe their baby.
Movement	Rocking and dancing and bouncing are instinctive responses to baby's developmental needs – and can be great fun!

If you ever doubt what a good job you're doing, ask yourself whose child you would swap your own for. (Giles 1997)

TIME FOR REFLECTION

Look back at the parents' agenda drawn up at the start of the antenatal course. Have you covered everything they asked for? Ask them to check the list with you, to show how important you think their needs are.

As you try the activities, you will adopt them wholesale, modify or reject them. Attend workshops and study days to get more ideas and look in books and websites to get new inspiration. Different exercises suit different groups – and different educators. Evaluate their usefulness using the methods described in the final chapter of this book.

WHERE NOW?

At present, only 50% of women are attending antenatal classes and even fewer men. Teenage parents and those on low incomes are hard to reach. There is a need for more flexibility in provision and more individualised educational approaches (Hames 1997). May (2000) describes the success of non-traditional antenatal classes: drop-in sessions, sessions targeted at particular stages of pregnancy, one-off workshops on specific topics. In addition, we should be looking at ways to extend contact with parents, so that antenatal education becomes *perinatal* education. Postnatal discussion groups or unstructured drop-in sessions can be planned.

Excellent information for perinatal educators is given in Chapters 10 and 17 of Page (2000). There is an urgent need for more collaboration, not just between midwives and health visitors, as Underdown (1998) suggests, but between health professionals and qualified adult educators.

KEY POINTS

God intended motherhood to be a relay race. Each generation would pass the baton on to the next. But the baton has been fumbled. So, it's our job – yours and mine – to pick it up. We have to do more than follow in our mother's footsteps; we have to ... rediscover the lost art of mothering. (Mary Pride, in Saavedra 1992:220)

Programmed by millions of years of evolution, babies are designed to get what they need from their parents. Parents too have developed to love and nurture their children. A baby, however, is fully in tune with its primitive instincts; many modern parents are not.

The work of the educator is to re-attune parents to these instincts, to give them the confidence to follow them and to enable them to acquire the many additional skills they need to cope with being a family in a far from primitive society.

REFERENCES

Belsky J, Kelly J 1994 The transition to parenthood. How a first child changes a marriage. Vermillion, London

Corwin A 1998 Integrating preparation for early parenting into childbirth education. Part I – a curriculum. Journal of Perinatal Education 7(4): 26–32

Corwin A 1999 Integrating preparation for early parenting into childbirth education. Part II – a study. Journal of Perinatal Education 8(1): 22–28

Daines J, Daines C, Graham B 1993 Adult learning, adult teaching. Continuing Education Press, Nottingham

England P, Horowitz R 1998 Birthing from within. An extra-ordinary guide to childbirth preparation. Partera Press, Albuquerque, NM

Giles A 1997 In the wrong. New Generation: Journal of the NCT June: 14–15

Hames P 1997 Parents' needs. New Generation Digest: Journal of the NCT (suppl) June: 5–7

Holmes K, Newburn M 1999 NCT services – birth, becoming a mother and baby feeding. New Generation Digest October: 18–20

Knox C 1997 Having it all. New Generation: Journal of the NCT June: 12

Larkin V, Butler M 2000 The implications of rest and sleep following childbirth. British Journal of Midwifery 8(7): 438–442

Leach P 1999 When babies are wakeful, who has the sleeping problem? Professional Care of Mother and Child 9(5): 117–120

Leonhardt-Lupa M 1995 A mother is born. Preparing for motherhood during pregnancy. Bergin and Garvey, Westport, Conn

May R 2000 Preparing for birth and a new baby. Practising Midwife 3(7): 44–45

Nolan ML 1997 Antenatal education: failing to educate for parenthood. British Journal of Midwifery 5(1): 21–26

Nolan ML 1998 Antenatal education: a dynamic approach. Baillière Tindall: Edinburgh

Nolan ML 1999 Antenatal education: past and future agendas. Practising Midwife 2(3): 24–27

Ockenden J 2000 After the birth is over: rest and support for new mothers. Practising Midwife 3(11): 10–13

O'Driscoll M 1998 Midwives discover sex. Practising Midwife 2(6): 32–33

Page LA (ed) 2000 The new midwifery. Science and sensitivity in practice. Churchill Livingstone, London

Polomeno V 2000 The Polomeno family intervention framework for perinatal education – preparing couples for the transition to parenthood. Journal of Perinatal Education 9(1): 31–48

Priest J, Schott J 1991 Leading antenatal classes: a practical guide. Butterworth Heinemann, Oxford

Pugh G, De'Ath E, Smith C 1994 Confident parents, confident children: policy and practice in parent education and support. National Children's Bureau, London

Raphael-Leff J 1991 Psychological processes of childbearing. Chapman and Hall, London

Robinson-Walsh D 1996 From couple to family. New Generation: Journal of the NCT December: 10–11

Rogers J 1989 Adults learning, 3rd edn. Open University Press, Milton Keynes

Saavedra BW 1992 Meditations for new mothers. Aquarian/Thorsons, London

Schott J 1994 The importance of encouraging women to think for themselves. British Journal of Midwifery 2(1): 3–4

Sherr L 1995 The psychology of pregnancy and childbirth. Blackwell Science, Oxford

Smith A 1998 Influences from the past. New Generation Digest September: 2–3

Underdown A 1998 The transition to parenthood. British Journal of Midwifery 6(8): 508–511

6 Parenting education for men

Nina Smith

INTRODUCTION

Society has a complicated view on men as fathers. On the one hand, they are judged to be not supportive enough of their partners, not sufficiently involved with their children or, if they are involved, aggressive or abusive. Fathers seem to get a consistently bad press (Lloyd 1995). On the other hand, there is much less consideration for them adjusting to a new role as a parent than there is for women becoming mothers. Jordan (1990) found that men were in a strangely ambiguous situation when it came to impending fatherhood – expected to be more involved and caring but with little available to help them be so. Since then, the issues of fatherhood have gained much more attention. Government policy sees working with men-as-fathers as high priority. In practice, however, it may be harder to fathom the most appropriate and acceptable ways for this work to take place.

As we start to move into the 21st century there seems to have been no other time in history when everyone has been so worried about males and the male role. Concerns expressed by politicians, education experts, psychiatrists, family-centred organisations and media pundits have popularised the debate. There is concern about boys underachieving at school, about high suicide rates amongst young men and about men generally losing their way, including in their role as fathers. Non-involvement of fathers has led to a lack of good male role models for boys. This in turn has led to boys growing into men who continue the pattern of non-resident fatherhood, lack of involvement and failure to model for the next generation of boys. A worrying cycle has been set up which it is hard to break (Clare 2000).

Pugh & De'Ath (1984) and Pugh et al (1994) called for a 'lifecycle' approach to parenting education which would begin in school and extend right through to grandparenthood. Within this sensible thesis, which is long overdue for implementation, much comment was made about men becoming fathers and the need to ease their transition to parenthood by starting to prepare boys for their future role and allowing men to fully participate in antenatal and postnatal education and support.

WORKING WITH FATHERS

Within the field of education for parenthood, fathers are a particularly topical issue. However, it would be wrong not to acknowledge at the outset the difficulties which anyone working with men to support learning about fathering may encounter.

Making false assumptions

It is easy to make assumptions about men's behaviour and the role and remit of fathers and to forget that individual fathers work out their roles in many different ways. Ralph LaRossa provided a thought-provoking angle when writing of the:

> *culture of fatherhood* (specifically the shared norms, values and beliefs surrounding men's parenting) and the *conduct of fatherhood* (what fathers do, their paternal behaviours). The distinction between culture and conduct is worth noting because although it is often assumed that the culture and conduct of a society are in sync., the fact is that many times the two are not synchronised at all. (LaRossa 1988:451)

The way men work out their role as fathers is influenced by a whole range of cultural, ethnic and socioeconomic factors which cannot be ignored. Anyone trying to offer parenting education needs to be prepared to work with, not against, these factors.

Funding

After many years during which the father's role in child development was denied, it is now considered to be a key influence in the emotional, academic and social well-being of both boys and girls (Ryan 2000:1). Government funding tends to be directed towards projects which make an explicit link between the active involvement of fathers and the improved welfare of children. (Not all agencies are totally happy with this. Too much emphasis on the role of fathers can stigmatise children who, through no choice of their own, have no father in their lives.) However, helping men to learn about being a parent often demands great sensitivity to the complex circumstances of fathers' lives and a deep understanding of local conditions. It can be hard to sustain the type of groups which the government particularly favours. Lack of funding is a reason why some fathers' groups have folded, even though they had much potential for success.

Image of groups

The ideas that both women and men have about groups for parents can present obstacles to learning. The image of men-only groups is particularly negative. A survey by the Institute of Public Policy Research which evaluated a number of such groups found that the men admitted to some anxiety about who else would attend, even when the individual concerned felt motivated to go to a group.

> Certainly, most of the fathers in this study reported feeling uneasy about coming to their initial meeting. One described standing outside the family centre and waiting to see what kinds of men participated in the fathers'

project before deciding to join the group himself. Nevertheless, facilitators often noted that once the ice is broken and an element of trust established, fathers readily relate to each other in ways supposedly only characteristic of women. (Longstaff 2000: 38)

My own research into antenatal classes and the transition to fatherhood carried out in 1996 produced mixed responses to the idea of men-only sessions (Smith 1999c). The men I interviewed who had not enjoyed their classes could see no benefit in having a class to themselves, presumably thinking that it would end up as irrelevant and sometimes boring, as they had found the shared classes. Those who had got a lot from their classes were much happier to think there might be more on offer just for them. But even those who felt a men-only session would be a good idea were concerned that to attend themselves might be detrimental to their self-image and to their image within their peer group. What sort of men would attend such classes – would they be odd in some way? Too 'alternative'? Too 'New Age'? Too different from how they saw themselves? Might the men who attended such a group be somehow 'unmanly'? It had been a huge relief to the respondents I interviewed in my study to discover that the other male participants in their antenatal classes were identical to themselves in background and had similar worries.

All the research and experience cited in this chapter underlines that men can get as much from educational/support groups as women. Yet the difficulty of getting men to attend groups can be demoralising for a highly motivated health professional or community worker, as Denise Barna revealed in her account of setting up a fathers' group in Sunderland (1995). Tenacity and commitment are required. Assumptions made by agencies which could set up a referral also contribute to men staying away from groups which might help and support them. David Bartlett (Bartlett & Plows 1998), writing the report on NEWPIN's Fathers' Support Group of 1997–98, observes that agencies 'presented an image of fathers being unwilling to make use of services' and therefore did not refer them to NEWPIN. The reality was that men were wary because they did not expect to be supported as fathers. Once they had been contacted, encouraged and *followed up proactively by NEWPIN* (my italics) a different picture emerged, with motivation and commitment developing.

Appropriate methods

Attending groups takes a high degree of motivation. Some men would never feel motivated to seek out a group or even attend one that had been recommended. So it is important to think laterally and appreciate that education for parenthood can be delivered in different ways. At present, the numbers attending men's groups are small. It may be that, in the context within which you work, groups for couples are more appropriate than groups for men only. If men come to parenting education at all, the most obvious starting point will be antenatal classes, attending with their pregnant partner. Pregnancy, according to Chalmers & McIntyre (1994), is 'the ideal teachable moment' because it is a time of great receptivity and openness to new ways of thinking since, implicitly, everything is becoming new. Changing the formats of antenatal courses may be a necessary next step so that some of the teaching occurs *after* the baby is born, thus maintaining continuity and enhancing men's perception of the relevance of classes to their needs.

I am using the term 'education' very loosely. Support and education in the field of parenting overlap and merge constantly and 'education' is a word which many participants in, and facilitators of, parents' groups would certainly not use. In many cases, the educational process means peers supporting each other as each individual learns to grow into a new role – surely the oldest form of education there can be. Work with individuals and individual families can include education for parenthood even when this is not the overt reason for the contact between health professional and client. For some fathers, it is this method which will be the most effective – and it should not be undervalued.

In this chapter I look at working with men's groups, working with couples and working with individuals. Much could be written on them all but I present a few models on which to base work with men so that you can apply them as seems appropriate in the circumstances in which you encounter fathers. I offer some practical ideas for ensuring that men's needs are met in mixed gender groups and a few thoughts on working with individual men. I hope to generate an interest in an important subject and encourage you to investigate further.

Some of the groups I refer to ran only for a short period but that does not mean that they were a failure as a forum for education and support. Others are schemes which are only just beginning. A lot of experiments are taking place and it is currently difficult to pin down exactly what the best approaches might be.

MEN'S GROUPS

Although education and support programmes for fathers and specialised work with young men are a notable phenomenon of current parenthood education, groups for men do have an older history. Such groups were part of the developments in education for parenthood of the early part of the last century. When the first 'School for Mothers' was set up in London in 1907 for the education of 'good' mothers, it also included a bureau to give advice to fathers and ran 'evening conferences' for men to teach fathers their family duties. Dr Grantly Dick-Read ran classes in and around London, in the 1920s, for expectant fathers to help them support their wives and bond with their babies. These were started at the request of *men's* organisations. Men themselves saw a need and took steps to address that need. Although the style and content of Dick-Read's classes would probably now be considered patronising and inappropriate, it may be time for the concept of a man running antenatal classes for expectant fathers to be revisited.

The changes in society over the last 50 years have obliged men to try to work out their role as fathers in complex circumstances where bland, uniform solutions are not the answer. The way fathers' groups are organised today is diverse and any educator seeking to start up a group has many options to choose from. Some groups are more formal and facilitated; others are informal, unstructured and unfacilitated. In others, a group is started by a facilitator with the participants subsequently taking over. Many of these groups have small numbers. Those which are most popular, or whose participants are most determined to keep them going, tend to have some unifying theme which may arise out of the fathering role but also goes beyond it to include issues which affect men's lives in other ways. The theme might be interest in a particular activity; a strong commitment to campaigning; a need for discussion, education and support on a problem area associated with self, partner or child; health issues or child development.

FINDING A FOCUS

Although some groups will include mothers as well, for this section I want to look primarily at the men-only and father-and-baby/child groups.

BOX 6.1	*Some formats for fathers' groups*
	■ Father-and-baby sessions on Saturday mornings (babies up to 1 year) ■ Father support groups in the workplace – antenatal and postnatal ■ Informal groups following on from antenatal courses ■ Groups targeted at particular groups, e.g. black fathers; young fathers; sufferers from, or supporters of, those with postnatal depression; lone fathers; non-resident fathers; gay fathers ■ Drop-in sessions for fathers and their children

Deciding on the focus of a fathers' group seems to be an essential first step. The examples in the IPPR survey (Longstaff 2000) tend to cater for men who have very particular issues to deal with in their parenting role: for example, lone fathers, non-resident fathers, gay fathers. However, the report overall looks at a much wider spectrum, describing groups which fall into four categories: 'recreational, educational, therapeutic or campaigning'. Illuminating insights are given into the success or otherwise of the fathers' groups. The shared situation seems to be a factor in keeping a group running, although some of the groups are small, with a regular attendance of about four, and some have had great difficulties, particularly with funding. Important in the ethos of these groups is that they enable men to share the pleasures and fun that they gain from being fathers as well as helping them to learn how to deal with the problems.

The report concludes that:

> . . . whilst they are not the sole solution, fathers' groups constitute an important means of empowering men to bring about change in their own lives and in so doing push back the margins of modern fatherhood. (Longstaff 2000:59)

The scope for specifically targeted groups is wide; for example, groups for men coping either with their own or their partner's postnatal depression. Postnatal depression gets a lot of publicity and it is a topic about which expectant and new fathers can feel worried and uninformed. In my own research, postnatal depression emerged as an important subject for a men-only antenatal session (Smith 1998, 1999c). Newburn & MacMillan (1998), in the NCT/RCM New Fathers' Survey, found men wanted more information and support in this area.

Singh & Newburn (2000:27) report that, in their survey, 63% of the men about to become fathers wanted information about postnatal depression compared with 59% of women.

Sullivan-Lyons (1999), who has a particular concern for men suffering from postnatal depression, suggests the possibility of setting up groups specifically for men during the time of the transition to parenthood. The prevalence of postnatal depression in men is recognised to a greater extent now, with its cause attributed in some cases to the partner's postnatal depression and in others, to difficulties in adjustment to fatherhood (Ballard et al 1994).

There is also scope for special groups in the workplace. The demands of work affect the amount of contact a father has with his child and are bound to have an influence on how involved he is as a father (Garbarino 1993). Singh & Newburn (2000: Section 3.3) report that two-fifths of the fathers surveyed found that employment impinged on the amount of time they could spend with their babies. Starting groups within the workplace to support and inform fathers is one suggested way to help address the very real conflicts that can arise within families over fathers who are too preoccupied with work to get to know their children (Snarey 1993). Such groups would not solve the problems but would raise awareness and give support. Like some of the other groups referred to below, there could also be a strong health education element.

Clare (2000) cites plenty of research throughout his book to show that fathers are more stable and ultimately more productive employees and greater contributors to the community than men who are not fathers. It is therefore worthwhile for an employer to take care of them *as fathers*. The fact that Clare's book is entitled *On Men: Masculinity in Crisis* and examines closely the enormous problems and challenges facing men in contemporary society powerfully makes the point that things need to be done differently. Workplace groups would be a bold venture. When fathers are working extraordinarily long hours (and it is common knowledge that British men work the longest hours in Europe) it may be hard to justify taking time out of work to attend a support group. However, a once-monthly lunchtime session, for example, may be something to think about. The models do not exist yet but the National Childbirth Trust is hoping to set up education/support for parenthood in workplaces for both women and men through corporate employee membership. The intention is to be flexible, responding to what parents require.

SOME MODELS OF GROUPS FOR FATHERS

Groups come in all sizes and types. Education for parenthood is such a fluid concept that it can be poured into many different moulds and still be effective. Different groups have been tried in all sorts of locations. A few examples are given below.

The NEWPIN Fathers' Support Programme

- Run in collaboration with other agencies
- Held in a day centre

- Accessible to any man needing support in caring for a child under the age of 18
- Wide range of groups: includes young and black dads; fathers with new babies; also has groups for men and women together
- Runs programmes of different duration, e.g. some programmes last 8 weeks, some 9 months
- Choice of timing – weekdays or weekends
- Run initially as a pilot project and developed into a continuing programme after positive evaluation.

American group

Peterson & Walls (1991) reported an American programme for fathers and their babies up to 1 year old. The main theme was enhancing child development by involving the father but the group also addressed wider issues.

- Held on Saturday mornings
- Content semi-structured – varied depending on the stated needs of the fathers
- First-time attenders primarily interested in baby's physical and personality development and discussing changes in relationship with partner
- Fathers returning for subsequent sessions wanted new information about the baby's current state of growth
- Format: discussion and hands-on experience. Wide range of subjects discussed: the father's role in the development of the child; changed relationships with partners; and particular situations such as mothers suffering from postnatal depression or mothers wanting to return to work
- Evaluation of facilitators: fathers' sense of the significance of their role in their child's development bolstered; stronger attachment to the baby; recognition of uniqueness of their contribution; increasing confidence in parenting skills. BUT the attenders were primarily middle-class fathers who were highly motivated. Speculated that sessions would be harder to deliver to fathers 'who are not motivated, do not have a basic positive self-image as a father and do not have some basic parenting skills'.

Lincolnshire group

Vince Ion (2000) wrote of a successful group he ran in Lincolnshire for first-time fathers and their babies aged 10–12 weeks. The additional focus here was on men's health.

- One-off session run every other month over a period of 16 months
- Held out of normal working hours
- Held in the back room of a pub (free of charge)
- Invitations sent (with 60% attendance from those invited)
- Negotiation to allow a drink and a cigarette (benefit of using a pub) but no smoking during the session itself

■ Format: session in two parts:
   1. issues around fatherhood (triggered by the facilitator sharing his own experiences)
   2. issues of men's health (including coronary heart disease, cancer, mental health, accidents, sexual health)
■ Evaluation from men was very positive; they wanted further sessions.

Barna's group

This group for unemployed fathers and their children was co-facilitated successfully by a man and a woman. Barna's group, like the Lincolnshire group, also illustrates how useful these initiatives can be for health education: the men involved were more inclined to use the health services for themselves and their children as a result of going to the group. Another interesting aspect of this particular group is that, although sport was intended to be part of the agenda, the men themselves quickly revealed that they preferred to spend the time discussing parenthood and health-related issues.

FATHERS, SONS AND POTENTIAL FATHERS

There is work going on with young men and boys too, the 'potential fathers' (a term used by the Coram Family Moyenda Project) who need good modelling for adult life, including fatherhood. It is important not to forget the lifecycle approach. Both fathers and sons benefit from greater involvement with each other. In the IPPR survey (Longstaff 2000), the section on the National NEW-PIN Fathers' Support Project states:

> NEWPIN stresses that both parents have an important role to play in children's development; indeed, they argue that the failure of men to develop close, positive relationships with their children can have devastating effects on the whole family. (p. 47)

Lamb (1997), writing about fatherhood schemes in the US, observes: 'motivated men often complain that a lack of skills (exemplified by ignorance or clumsiness) prevents increased involvement and closeness' with their children. He maintains that the necessary skills can be learnt through 'formal skill-development programs' but also 'more informally through involvement in activities that children and fathers enjoy doing together'.

■ The YMCA and Care for the Family project, known as 'Dads and Lads', promotes opportunities for fathers and sons, or mentors and boys, to play sport together. Clare's examination of the research (2000) would support the view that fathers being actively involved with their sons (and also their daughters) is one of the best ways of ensuring the well-being of the parents of the future. The YMCA gives good information and support to those wanting to set up such a project. In its introductory pack, guidelines for running a project suggest that a variety of sports be offered, preferably not 'overtly competitive'. But it also suggests that leaders listen to the participants, include requested activities and give information about related activities, such as talks on parenting issues. After attending four or five sessions, the dads are invited to attend a basic parenting course.

- Potential fathers of African, Afro-Caribbean and South Asian origin, are also a focus of work by the Coram Family Moyenda Project. The project sees its work not as related directly to fathering but to gender issues within the community it serves. It offers workshops, seminars and courses for those working with, or planning to work with, men from the particular cultures in which it specialises.

- The Black Men's Forum in Leeds is another example of an organisation working with males of African descent which focuses on the entirety of men's lives, with fatherhood and potential fatherhood as one aspect.

- NEWPIN's Fathers' Centre is developing a project for 'teenage boys who are likely to become fathers over the next few years'. This is in partnership with other agencies and plans to offer groups looking at such issues as self-esteem, personal growth, self-awareness and masculinity, life skills, health and sexuality, as well as responsible parenthood and the links between them all.

- PIPPIN (Parents in Partnership Parent Infant Network) has its own 'Investing in Fathers' project which is targeted at young fathers, under 25 years old, who are not living with their partner or baby, from pregnancy through to 4 months after the birth. The project intends to listen to these young men and find out what education and support will be most relevant for them.

The models I have picked out have been written up in detail or the organisations concerned are willing to share the experience of setting up and running these groups and the outcomes for participants. Details of how to find these reports and contact the organisations appear at the end of the chapter.

In addition, a whole range of fathers' groups has been set up across the country, many of them within the province of child protection. Examples of good practice are reported for the Department of Health by Mary Ryan in *Working with Fathers* (2000). This publication has useful information for those trying to set up groups and contact points for fathers, both resident and non-resident.

GROUPS FOR 'LOW-RISK' FATHERS

Close targeting of groups is an excellent way for support/education to be delivered to fathers with extra needs. But what about the men who would never attend such a group because they don't fit into the targeted category, those who would be considered 'low risk'? The majority of fathers are resident, will never come to the notice of child protection workers and do not present to any agency with particular problems. Nonetheless, they might gain enormously from sharing and developing parenting skills, offloading worries and stresses and enjoying the fun of fathering, to the benefit of their children and partners. The term 'low risk' I have taken from Parr's (1998) article in the BJM where she talks about the findings of the PIPPIN programme. She argues that 'low-risk' couples can still experience 'psychological distress' in adjusting to parenthood.

In my own study in 1996, I asked 18 fathers who had attended antenatal classes whether they would have liked postnatal classes. All the respondents fell into the low-risk category and for some the thought of more classes was unappealing, especially if they had a low opinion of their antenatal classes. For others there was mild interest and for quite a few, it seemed a necessary next step. I interviewed these men when their babies were aged between 4 and 13 weeks. Nine had attended NHS classes and nine National Childbirth Trust classes (see Box 6.2).

BOX 6.2	*Men's views on postnatal classes*

I'd have been interested in going. I wonder if there'd be time though, that's the problem, isn't it? Finding the time. 'Cos there's so little time . . . you've got the new baby . . . you just want to be at home all the time and when you're not at home you have to be at work.

Postnatal classes? Oh yes, definitely. I'd have signed on the dotted line.

It's interesting to get together and talk. I think it's a great shame that it all shuts down after birth.

Yeah, postnatal classes would be really good. 'Cos you'd get a chance just to have a month or whatever to settle down, and then you could raise all the things that had cropped up. 'Cos *loads* of things crop up.

I would certainly have thought it would be very useful to go on one or two postnatal classes with other couples who'd recently had babies and have some sort of structured discussions as couples.

What more could the antenatal classes have done to prepare us for parenthood? Would any of it have sunk in when we were really focused on this birth? . . . A lot of it may not have done. We would have felt quite favourable to the idea of postnatal classes.

I think I would have been unlikely to sign up for another course of classes 'cos of your natural alienation from anything to do with classes and school, you know.

I wouldn't have sort of really liked that idea . . . the midwives came round to the house once a day and I think that's really sufficient.

I think they would be very useful . . . it's a very, very strange situation to find yourself in, even when you've gone to antenatal classes . . . this small, fragile baby . . . you don't know what it does and why it does things and whether it's happy or unhappy . . . education makes it easier.

Several things emerge from these comments:

- the mixed nature of the responses
- those who like the idea of postnatal parenting classes think very much in terms of attending as couples. Like the antenatal classes, postnatal classes are to be shared with a partner, reflecting the partnership of parenthood
- a hint that continuity from the ante to the postnatal period is valuable
- those who are not keen cite lack of time and lack of interest in 'school' type activities.

Managing time and preferring to be at home with the baby rather than out at a group seem perfectly valid reasons for not attending. Lack of enthusiasm for 'education' in the generally understood sense of the word is common, as experienced educators will not need to be told. Current fathers' groups are working on a very different model from formal education. Postnatal sessions need to be as flexible as possible. When time is at a premium, the facility for dropping in and out is crucial and applies to both men and women attending such sessions.

WORKING WITH COUPLES

An obvious starting point for parenting education is the antenatal course which is a well-established system and supported by a considerable amount of expertise. Although men frequently come to antenatal classes because they see this as a way of supporting their partner, when given the opportunity they will often reveal that they have a personal agenda too, even if it seems hard to articulate. This agenda often revolves around the demands of parenthood, becoming a father and practicalities of babycare just as much as around pregnancy and birth (Nolan 1994, Smith 1999a-c). Singh & Newburn's study (2000) of men from varied social, economic and ethnic backgrounds shows that, before the birth, over half the men wanted either 'a great deal' or 'quite a lot' of information about life with a new baby (Section 2.2).

The need for education and support continues throughout the transition to parenthood. Learning before the birth does not mean that the same individuals have no need to re-learn or reinforce skills and gather new knowledge later on. Given that it seems easier to attract men into groups when they are *expectant* fathers, it may make sense to link the period before and after the birth by splitting a course into ante and postnatal sections or by following up an antenatal course with some postnatal sessions. Some National Childbirth Trust courses are now structured in this way so that they can address postnatal needs when they are no longer an unknown quantity and education therefore has more meaning. Continuity from the ante to the postnatal period is ensured for the couples involved. Helping fathers as well as mothers to learn 'on the job' makes sense.

The PIPPIN programmes, which concentrate on parent–parent and parent–infant relationships to ease the adjustment to family life, operate in the same fashion. Couples can attend both ante and postnatally, enabling them to learn about the practical and emotional impact of parenting in a safe group which supports them through the transition to parenthood and beyond. The courses are discussion based and aim to give parents an opportunity to learn about themselves and their babies. PIPPIN aims to incorporate its methodology into programmes which are being run by professionals or voluntary workers.

SOME PRACTICAL SUGGESTIONS

Some topics to ensure that the needs of expectant fathers are met within mixed gender antenatal classes are suggested in Box 6.3. However, the topics will be just as relevant for groups run after the birth of the baby.

BOX 6.3	*Parenting issues for mixed gender groups (before and after birth)*

- Crying babies
- Sleeping and sleeping arrangements
- Feeding babies – practicalities and feelings
- Practical babycare
- Balancing work and home
- Postnatal depression
- Changed lifestyle
- Changed relationships – between partners, with the extended family and friends
- Support systems
- Baby behaviour and development
- Handling anger with babies and small children
- Knowing if the baby is ill and what to do
- Wider family health issues
- Fathers and sons

Men's reasons for attending classes are linked to both the ante and postnatal periods. The transition to parenthood needs to be seen by parents and educators alike as a single, continuous process.

Men attend classes:

- to demonstrate support for their partner
- to show commitment to future care of their partner and child
- to gain knowledge
- to define a role (Smith 1998, 1999a,c)

You can incorporate these into aims for parenting education for men attending antenatal and postnatal courses (see Box 6.4).

It is very important for men to feel as safe in a parents' group as the women, be it before or after the birth. They will not share views or absorb information if they do not feel properly integrated and welcome in the group. If you are female, you need to be very aware that you are running a mixed-gender group: don't lead it as if it were only for women. It is important to keep in mind that:

- men need to have *their* worries, fears and aspirations acknowledged
- men need to be addressed and treated as equals
- single-sex group work and single-sex teaching are empowering for men.

Don't embarrass the men or reinforce the 'man-as-spare-part' attitude by making or endorsing remarks which stereotype men in this way. You might like to explore the idea of parallel sessions for men only.

SINGLE-SEX GROUP WORK

Within mixed-gender groups, both before and after the birth, single-sex group work can be an invaluable tool. In my own research (Smith 1999c) it was one of the ways suggested by the men themselves for better addressing fathers'

BOX 6.4	*Course aims*

Antenatally	Postnatally
■ Give expectant fathers an arena to demonstrate support for their partners and commitment to the future family.	■ Provide new fathers with an opportunity to debrief their experience of labour and birth in a safe environment and assess its emotional impact.
■ Offer men an equal opportunity to learn about pregnancy, labour, birth and early parenting.	■ Enable new fathers to learn, with their partners, about day-to-day life as a parent, baby development and family health issues, and acquire practical skills.
■ Empower men in their role as father by giving them information and practical skills for the postnatal period and raise awareness of the impact a new baby has on relationships, lifestyle, emotions and attitudes of both mothers and fathers.	■ Empower men in their new role as father by providing a safe and non-judgemental environment in which they can share the experiences and emotions of parenting with their peers.
■ Provide a safe, non-judgemental environment in which men can share thoughts and feelings on becoming a father.	■ Provide a supportive network of parents for the future.

needs. Sullivan-Lyons (1999), referring to the study 'Men Becoming Fathers' where the men researched had been to NHS classes, observes:

> Both men and women indicated that the men did not ask many questions at these classes, mainly because of not wishing to appear ignorant about pregnancy and labour, but also because they felt embarrassed to do so. (p. 238)

Looking particularly at the mental health of new fathers, she says:

> It may be that antenatal classes organised for the benefit of pregnant women are not the most appropriate setting for men to ask questions and talk about any worries they have about the pregnancy, labour or becoming a father . . . Caregivers must be wary of their efforts to include fathers becoming tokenistic. (p. 239)

Too much single-sex group work can become heavy-handed and cause resentment of enforced male bonding. It's always useful for any female facilitator to be mindful of Seel's memorable description of how much men dislike antenatal classes where they feel 'matronized' by the females present (Seel 1987, p. 47). No doubt the same would be true in postnatal groups. Sullivan-Lyons (1999) suggests parallel sessions for fathers, where they may feel less intimidated by the presence of women – a solution which might work extremely well if two educators work together. Involving men in the facilitation of such sessions is something that would be worth developing.

Allowing expectant fathers some time with the educator away from the women, preferably in a separate room, is highly productive. Questions usually come plentifully, including those they don't wish to ask in front of the women because they don't want to frighten them. Men have their own anxieties which need to be either allayed or talked about in an open, adult, honest manner. Single-sex group work is a technique that can be applied just as usefully to post-natal groups.

BOX 6.5	*Single-sex formats*
■ The same discussion topic for groups of the same gender with feedback ■ Discussion topics for men *not* fed back to the large group. There is no need for all discussion to be reported back; allow some privacy ■ Time spent with a visiting experienced father – with a wide open agenda ■ Single-sex teaching group – time in a class where the educator spends time only with the fathers ■ Men-only group – a class totally for men.	

You might like to consider running an antenatal class for men only. This is not a new idea. A report from America in the 1980s showed that such a class, which included practical babycare, led by one male and one female facilitator, could be highly successful. The class was incorporated into programmes in both Milwaukee and Delaware (Taubenheim & Silbernagel 1988). Participants were not necessarily all first-time fathers and the learning that occurred because of the presence of experienced fathers was apparently considerable. The benefits of expectant and new fathers learning from more experienced fathers are regularly reported in successful schemes to help men learn about parenthood.

You could usefully draw on Anthony Clare's book (2000) *On Men: Masculinity in Crisis* for triggers for group discussion in men-only classes. Clare sets out a modified and expanded form of a table used in the Government of South Australia's recent 'Six Ways to Be a Better Dad' campaign, published by the Office for Families and Children, Southern Australia. It covers the areas of role modelling, work and family, caring, partnerships and spending time with children. Steve Biddulph's 'Five Fathering Essentials' in his book *Raising Boys* (1997) has a great deal to say that would be thought provoking in a men's group discussing bringing up boys. Box 6.6 is a précis to give you some ideas for raising key issues.

WORKING WITH INDIVIDUALS

So far I have been looking at men attending parenting groups but education and support come in many forms. Groups are not for every parent. The IPPR report (Longstaff 2000) makes this point also.

> . . . it is certainly the case that some men, whilst keen to become more involved in their children's upbringing, do not want to do so via membership of a fathers' group. Illustrating this point, a recent large-

---

| **BOX 6.6** | *Five Fathering Essentials (based on Biddulph 1997:14-15)* |

- Start early. Includes being involved in the pregnancy; being at the birth; getting involved with babycare; using weekends and holidays to get 'immersed with your child'.
- Make time. Includes taking a hard look at careers which take up 55 or 60 hours a week; problems created for sons by fathers not being around enough; making time to play and have fun with children.
- Be demonstrative. Includes hugging, holding, wrestling games, cuddling children; benefits for boys from such play with their fathers; reading stories, sitting together and listening to music with children; telling them how 'great, beautiful, creative and intelligent they are'.
- Lighten up. Includes enjoying children; having fun together with no pressure to achieve but not necessarily 'racing around' – also walks, games and conversation, 'time just to be'; encouraging sons to help in the home; teaching continuously.
- Heavy down. Includes 'calm but definite' discipline; being involved in decisions, supervising homework and housework; talking to partner and parenting as a team.

---

scale survey of Australian fathers found that the majority of men are concerned about their future roles as fathers, want to spend more time with their children and would seek parenting support, but that only 15% of men would consider joining a fathers' group (Russell et al 1999). It should not be supposed, however, that this reluctance to join groups is solely characteristic of fathers. Parenthood is a private business; many women are similarly disinclined to participate in public parenting programmes. (p. 39)

Both antenatally and postnatally midwives and health visitors have wonderful opportunities to educate while supporting couples and individuals in hospital and through home and hospital visits. The challenge is to see these encounters as opportunities for education as well as healthcare and to include men as well as women. Lester & Moorsom (1997) urged midwives not to see the health of women and babies in isolation from that of other members of a family unit. They rightly observe that the father is 'an integral member' of that family unit and that midwives should extend their practice to include support for men during the transition to parenthood in order to maintain the physical and emotional health of all concerned.

It is good news to read in Singh & Newburn (2000) that two-thirds of men found that they were given as much attention by midwives in the first 10 days after the birth of their baby as they required in terms of answering questions and taking notice of their views and wishes. But the bad news is that one in 10 said they were never given the chance to ask questions or express their opinions, with men under 20 most likely to find that midwives did not explain to them what to expect from a new baby. The opportunities for informal education are there but it takes a conscious effort to include fathers when for decades so much emphasis has been on mother–infant relationships.

Trevelyan (1996), reporting on the 1996 IPPR conference, looks at the exclusion of fathers by health visitors from involvement with their children because the focus is so much on mothers. Ion (2000) concludes:

Not all health professionals will feel comfortable about addressing issues surrounding fatherhood. However, it is vital that health visitors devise ways of engaging with fathers at an early stage. (p. 46)

A recommendation from their health visitor may send a lot of couples to parenting groups who would otherwise have missed out. Health visitors are ideally placed to get classes going. Many do. The key question is – how to involve men?

BOX 6.7	*Key issues*

- Getting the timing right so that fathers can be included.
- Not making assumptions about whether certain individuals would or would not be likely candidates for groups – let *them* decide.
- Seeing the family as a whole; not isolating the father.
- Encouraging discussion of feelings and relationships in classes as well as practical issues.

EDUCATORS AND FACILITATORS

It is worthwhile thinking carefully about *who* is going to deliver education programmes or facilitate the setting up of a group. The models which are cited in this chapter show that variety is possible and desirable. There is no single correct way. Men running groups for men and also a male-female facilitation team both seem to work if the context is right. The NEWPIN evaluation of the 1997–98 Fathers' Support Group (Bartlett & Plows 1998) shows how very positive male and female co-facilitation can be. Men don't necessarily learn better from another man. So much depends on previous life and learning experiences.

However, men should certainly be encouraged to help each other. Arranging some contact for men with experienced fathers is enormously helpful both ante and postnatally. Educators may need to re-think their approach in this context and involve men much more in an educational role. Female educators, facilitators, discussion leaders (however you think of yourself) should consider what partnerships could be set up to ensure that education for parenthood caters properly for fathers. It may be necessary to examine and deal with personal prejudices and allow men to participate in the field of parenthood education far more than has hitherto been the norm. The men in my study talked constantly of 'the partnership of parenthood'. It may be time for a partnership of educators.

CONCLUSION

The official interest in helping men learn about parenthood is undeniable and the challenge this presents to educators is self-evident. Parenting education for men is a new field and educators will need to do a lot of listening and learning before anyone can confidently say which is the most appropriate way to deliver such education. Current experience in running fathers' groups is fragmented but the models are there. Much experience has been gained and many lessons learned from classes for expectant fathers. Those who are working with men's issues, as opposed to specifically fathering issues, also have a great deal of knowledge and expertise. An exchange of ideas seems sensible to move things on.

Approaches to looking after the *whole* family are urgently required. Men need to be considered as well as women and children. Men themselves want more consideration. The setting up of Fathers Direct to focus specifically on the needs of fathers and act as a resource for men and those working with men alike is indicative of a change of mood around family matters. Parenting education for women has always worked best when it is needs led, with those involved trying to respond to what individual women want to learn. The same is true of parenting education for men.

| KEY POINTS | However they behave, fathers, whether they be absent or present, are a significant part of the lives of most children in need and the research studies suggest that it is difficult to achieve optimal outcomes without including the man as at least the subject — if not an active participant — of professional deliberation. Engaging with fathers is not beyond the powers of individual practitioners. (Ryan 2000:76–77) |

REFERENCES

Ballard CG, Davis R, Cullen PC, Mohan RN, Dean C 1994 Prevalence of psychiatric morbidity in mothers and fathers. British Journal of Psychiatry 164 (6):782–788

Barna D 1995 Working with young men. Health Visitor 68 (5): 185–187

Bartlett D, Plows B 1998 Report on NEWPIN's Fathers' Support Group 1997–98. NEWPIN Fathers' Centre, London

Biddulph S 1997 Raising boys. Thorsons, London

Chalmers B, McIntyre J 1994 Do antenatal classes have a place in modern obstetric care? Journal of Psychosomatic Obstetrics and Gynaecology 15 (2):119–123

Clare A 2000 On men: masculinity in crisis. Chatto and Windus, London

Garbarino J 1993 Reinventing fatherhood: families in society. Journal of Contemporary Human Services 74 (1):51–54

Ion V 2000 Accessible health sessions for first-time fathers. Nursing Times 96 (12):46

Jordan P 1990 Labouring for relevance: expectant and new fatherhood. Nursing Research 39 (1):11–16

Lamb ME 1997 Fathers and child development: an introductory overview and guide. In: Lamb ME (ed) The role of the father in child development. John Wiley, New York, pp 1–18

LaRossa R 1988 Fatherhood and social change. Family Relations 37: 451–457

Lester A, Moorsom S 1997 Do men need midwives? Facilitating a greater involvement in parenting. British Journal of Midwifery 5 (13):678–681

Lloyd T 1995 Fathers in the media: an analysis of newspaper coverage of fathers. In: Moss P (ed) Father figures in the families of the 1990s. HMSO, Edinburgh, pp 41–51

Longstaff E 2000 Fathers figure: fathers' groups in family policy. Institute for Public Policy Research, London

Newburn M, MacMillan M 1998 Help, new dad emerging. Practising Midwife 1 (1):17–19

Nolan M 1994 Caring for fathers in antenatal classes. Modern Midwife 4 (2):25–28

Parr M 1998 A new approach to parent education. British Journal of Midwifery 6 (3):160–165

Peterson FL, Walls D 1991 Fatherhood preparation during childbirth education. International Journal of Childbirth Education 4 (6):38–39

Pugh G, De'Ath E 1984 The needs of parents: practice and policy in parent education. Macmillan Education, London

Pugh G, De'Ath E, Smith C 1994 Confident parents, confident children: policy and practice in parent education and support. National Children's Bureau, London

Russell G, Barclay L, Edgecombe G, Donovan J, Habib G, Pawson Q 1999 Fitting fathers into families. Commonwealth Department of Family and Community Services, Australia

Ryan M 2000 Working with fathers. Radcliffe Medical Press, Abingdon

Seel R 1987 The uncertain father. Gateway Books, Bath

Singh D, Newburn M 2000 Becoming a father: men's access to information and support about pregnancy, birth and life with a new baby. National Childbirth Trust, London

Smith NJ 1998 What role do antenatal classes play for men in their transition to fatherhood? Dissertation, University of East Anglia

Smith NJ 1999a Men in antenatal classes: teaching 'the whole birth thing'. Practising Midwife 2 (1):23–26

Smith NJ 1999b Antenatal classes and the transition to fatherhood: a study of some fathers' views Part I. MIDIRS Digest 9 (3):327–330

Smith NJ 1999c Antenatal classes and the transition to fatherhood: a study of some fathers' views Part II. MIDIRS Digest 9 (4):463–468

Snarey J 1993 How fathers care for the next generation – a four-decade study. Harvard University Press, Cambridge, Mass

Sullivan-Lyons J 1999 Men becoming fathers: 'Sometimes I wonder how I'll cope'. In: Clement S (ed) Psychological perspectives on pregnancy and childbirth. Churchill Livingstone, Edinburgh

Taubenheim AM, Silbernagel T 1988 Meeting the needs of expectant fathers. American Journal of Maternal/Child Nursing 13 (2):110–113

Trevelyan J 1996 Father's day. Health Visitor 69 (6):213

RESOURCES

Information on fathers' groups

- Project for unemployed men in Sunderland with responsibility as the main childcarer; male and female facilitator. Report by Barna (1995).
- Groups surveyed in detail by IPPR and reported by Longstaff (2000):
  Shildon Single Fathers' Group, County Durham
  Stonewall Gay Dads' Group, London
  Men United, Nottingham
  Man Enough, Oxford
  National NEWPIN Fathers' Support Project, London
  The survey also gives a very good general analysis of the running of groups for fathers. Available from IPPR (see Useful Addresses).
- NEWPIN's Fathers' Support Group 1997–98 in London. Report by Bartlett & Plows (1998). Available from NEWPIN (see Useful Addresses).
- The Coram Family Moyenda Project welcomes visitors who want to learn about their work. Appointments must be made in advance by phone (see Useful Addresses).
- PIPPIN runs courses for professionals and voluntary workers in the field of parenting education (see Useful Addresses).
- 'Dads and Lads' schemes run by the YMCA and Care for the Family, funded by the Home Office. Started in Plymouth and running in other parts of the country. The YMCA also produces a magazine called 'DAD'. Sends out 'Dads and Lads' pack to enquirers with a leaflet: 'Ten Steps to Setting Up a Group' (see Useful Addresses).
- Sessions for first-time fathers and their babies in Lincolnshire. Reported by Ion (2000).

Useful addresses

Black Men's Forum, Chapeltown Enterprise Centre, 231 Chapeltown Road,
Leeds LS7 3DX
Tel: 0113 262 6233
Fax: 0113 262 1274
Email: bmf@cec-resources.co.uk

Coram Family, 49 Mecklenburgh Square, London WCIN 2QA
Tel: 020 7520 0300

Coram Family Moyenda Project, address as above
Tel: 020 7520 0328
Fax: 020 7520 0301
Email: moyenda@coram.org.uk

Fathers Direct, Tamarisk House, 37 The Televillage, Crickhowell NP8 1BP
Tel: 01873 810515
Fax: 01873 810633
Email: mail@fathersdirect.org
On-line magazine for fathers: www.fathersdirect.com

Institute for Public Policy Research, 30 Southampton Street, London WC2
Tel: 020 7470 6100

National NEWPIN Fathers' Centre, The Amersham Centre, Inville Road,
London SE17 2HY
Tel: 020 7740 8997
Fax: 020 7740 8994

National Childbirth Trust, Alexandra House, Oldham Terrace, London
W3 6NH
Tel: 020 8992 2616
Fax: 020 8992 5929
Website: www.nctpregnancyandbabycare.com

PIPPIN, 48 Drapers Road, Leyton, London E15 2AY
Website: www.pippin.org.uk
'Investing in Fathers' project
Tel/Fax: 01438 364449
Email: john@pippin.org.uk

YMCA England, Dads and Lads Project, Dee Bridge House, 25–27 Lower
Bridge Street, Chester CH1 1RS
Tel: 01244 403090
Fax: 01244 315108
Email: dirk@parenting.ymca.org.uk; ahowie@themail.co.uk

7 Supporting young parents

Frances Hudson

INTRODUCTION

Young parents. What does that conjure up for you? What immediately springs to mind? Take a moment to think about it.

None of us can help making assumptions; we have our own ideas about 'teenage parents', 'schoolgirl mothers', etc. and we cannot help but have a view. Let us accept this. We tend to stereotype and we make judgements. We can't help it. But we can help what we do with these judgements and assumptions. When we wish to help anyone, the best thing to do with these is to leave them behind us and focus on the individual concerned. In negotiating with young people, this has to be the first rule, otherwise none of the rest will work.

Young people have less experience of life and they therefore have less understanding of the possible consequences of their actions. And yet they feel powerful, sometimes omnipotent. This is a particular quality of adolescence in our society. Adolescents often find it difficult to accept advice; they do not want to be told what they should do. If the young person is a parent, the difficulties for the professional helper are doubled. Not only does the parent require help and support but there is a child as well who needs a healthy start to life and this can best be provided by the mother (and the father if he is around).

A young mother's world may lack the support she needs; she may not have had good models of fulfilling and loving relationships; she may not have positive experiences of communication in her relationships. Our task is to help her learn to relate to and communicate lovingly with her child, which we call 'bonding'. In order for her to do this, we have to show her the greatest respect and attention. We can be for her a model of good communication and a meaningful relationship.

For the benefit of this chapter, let us define young parents as any mother (or father) from the age of 13 to 19. However, it must be conceded that this is not a homogeneous group, as a 13 year old is likely to be far less mature – physically, emotionally, intellectually – than a 19 year old. This needs to be understood in the following discussion of parenting skills for teenagers.

As health workers, our brief is to give mothers (and fathers if we get the chance) all the encouragement we can to become 'good-enough parents' and we do this by 'educating' them as best we can, given the constraints on our time and the young parents' receptiveness. It is worth unpacking this word 'educating'. It means 'drawing or leading out', as opposed to 'putting in', as in informing, advising, telling. The most effective education builds on the strengths, knowledge, potential and insights in the target audience, so that they will want to participate fully. And there is no doubt that many young mothers have considerable insight into their situation and are able to project beyond it, as Alison Hadley's book (1999) *Tough Choices* amply demonstrates.

> My advice to any young teenager planning on having a baby is to wait. It won't do you any harm. If you're going out with someone and they love you, then they'll wait. You should go and get a career, make sure you're in a steady, happy relationship and then, if it's what you both want, go for it. But remember it's an expensive and tiring business. If, like me, it's an accident, then do what your heart tells you . . . Do what you want to do because, at the end of the day, you're the one who has to live with the decision. Whatever your choice, make sure it's the right one. (Helen Tomlinson's story in Hadley 1999:59)

This chapter will look at specific strategies to make the best of the opportunities available to us for educating and supporting young parents. These strategies involve:

- examining our own responses to help and advice
- understanding relationships
- task-centred and person-centred approaches to helping
- monitoring our use of language
- demonstrating how to be with the child
- handling obstructive behaviour
- giving constructive feedback.

OUR OWN RESPONSES TO HELP AND ADVICE

It helps to take a little time to look honestly at our own reactions when someone comes along and tries to tell us how we might do things. If we feel we're being told off or criticised, we may react with resentment or sulk, get defensive or be angry. Criticism, valid or invalid, often feels threatening. If we feel under attack, whatever the advice being given, it is unlikely to be heeded.

So now to the young parent. I shall focus mainly on the mother from now on. What are her circumstances? We need to see each parent as an individual and be very careful not to think we know anything about her view of the world. We must not make assumptions about her parenting skills. We would take offence if anybody did this to us. It helps to remember that each individual we presume to help is the expert on her experience to date. What is important is to start where the parent is and build on what is already given.

When we were first parents, what did we already know and how did we learn to get parenting right? How many mistakes did we make? Who was there to back us up when things went wrong – or in case things went wrong? Anybody? How did we feel asking for and accepting help and support when we needed it? Did we, in fact, ask? Were we even aware that we needed help and support? And were there others around for this?

UNDERSTANDING RELATIONSHIPS

There is often conflict for a young mother: she wants to spoil her child on the one hand – give him more than he needs in material terms – and on the other, give him less than he needs in emotional terms. She is thus spoiling and punishing him at the same time, more than likely repeating negative patterns in her own upbringing. What is important is to help her understand what happened to her in the past and why, without apportioning blame. Blaming her parents will not help because they probably did the best for her that they could in the circumstances in which they found themselves. If a young mother can be helped to realise when she is inadvertently repeating the patterns of her own upbringing, she can move on from there. She may be able to work through her own childhood in a parenting group where other parents, from similar or different backgrounds, are also exploring how their own experience of being parented influences the way in which they are bringing up their children.

Recent research (Ingham et al 2000) has shown that young people who report that their parents 'were not there for them' were more likely to engage in early intercourse. This study controlled for other factors such as level of deprivation. When we think about how we learned our behaviour and attitudes, it becomes clear that our major task in helping young parents with their parenting skills is to encourage them to 'be there' for their own children. We can model this by being there for the young parents – giving them the love and attention they need, answering questions honestly and appropriately and admitting to ignorance if necessary! Young parents are able to be there for their children if they have had and preferably still have the experience of others being there for them. Their own parents supporting them with unconditional love is an obvious example; friends are an additional advantage. A good relationship with the baby's father helps enormously; sadly, this is not always in place for a young mother. The lack of a loving partner on whom she can rely for emotional and practical support (even if not for financial) is often a disappointment for her and possibly a confirmation of her experience of the world as a difficult and unloving place. This state of affairs does nothing for her self-esteem.

If there has never been anyone there for her, it is not surprising that a young mother has a chip on her shoulder and we should bear in mind that this is a defence mechanism, a coping strategy to deal with life. One of the reasons for her wanting a child of her own might be that she is trying to fill the need gap, thinking that a child will provide the love and attention she herself has missed.

TASK-CENTRED AND PERSON-CENTRED APPROACHES TO SUPPORT AND EDUCATION

In our concern to make sure that the child develops healthily and the mother learns the appropriate parenting skills to enable this to happen, we can often feel frustrated and a little judgemental. As professional educators or facilitators, we inevitably have our own agenda, a set of tasks to be addressed. It is not always easy to engage the interest of a young person whose pride in her new responsibilities may have worn off a little as she settles into a routine with her child. Rather than going straight for the task, some person-centred work is essential. By this, I don't simply mean asking how she is, how the night has been, whether her child . . .

It is a mistake to focus first and foremost on the practical tasks. These are easier to address since they engage the young mother in immediate and physical acts. Better but less easy is to engage the young mother on an emotional level and encourage her to open up about her situation and her view of the world. This person-centred aspect of our work is as important as teaching the practical tasks of parenthood.

MONITORING OUR USE OF LANGUAGE

I shall touch briefly on what kind of language works with young people already feeling vulnerable and possibly defensive, what doesn't work and why.

Questions come easily to us. However, they often sound as though we're being critical. It is better to try not asking questions. Closed questions are particularly problematic since they can sound judgemental; this is exactly what leads a young person to shut down and cease to take anything in. Since our job is to encourage the young mother to talk about how things are for *her*, as well as for her child, asking closed questions is unlikely to achieve this. Talking about how things are helps her to think through things at her own pace. Try telling her what she should do and we've lost her. Phrases such as 'If I were you . . .' and 'Why don't you . . . ?' have the same effect as closed questions. Open questions work better because they invite the other to talk about herself, knowing that we are interested. They require us to listen carefully to the responses and show close attention. How much do we need to know that will not be told to us willingly if we have built a good, trusting, mutually respectful relationship? Questions are best asked on a 'need to know' basis; even necessary knowledge can be obtained without asking direct questions if we try harder. We can use phrases which will have the effect of including the young mother and encourage her to take in our suggestions and benefit from our experience. These include:

- Let's have a go at mixing the feed/changing this nappy.
- I wonder how you're managing with mixing the feed/getting enough sleep/dealing with the tantrums.

The trick is to use 'I' statements (how something seems to us) rather than 'you', as these often come across as blaming and have the effect of shutting down the dialogue with the young mother. Also, lengthening sentences slightly can have a calming effect, giving her a feeling of being valued which enables her to respond thoughtfully.

Another way of engaging the attention and interest of the young mother is to let her see that we respect and value her ideas. This is achieved by letting her know that we're trying to see things from her point of view:

- From what you tell me . . .
- I get the impression that . . .
- It sounds as though . . .
- I get the feeling . . .

By inviting the young mother to comment on our understanding of her situation, we can avoid any misunderstanding or misinterpretation. Such uses of language encourage mothers and boost their self-esteem and confidence. We are also modelling communication strategies for the mother to take into her other relationships, with her baby or child, her parents, her partner. She will pick up positive messages (approval, appreciation, respect) from the way we talk to her and pass them along. If the mother feels OK, her child will thrive (Harris 1979). Unless the mother can express how she's feeling – her joys as well as her anxieties – and unless we pay great attention to her while she does this, she will not be open to learning. By being listened to, she feels confident and pleased and she can then transfer these good feelings to her child, interacting positively and lovingly with him. It is worth bearing in mind that for every negative a child receives, he needs four positives to redress the balance (Hamlin et al 1998).

DEMONSTRATING HOW TO BE WITH THE CHILD

There is a continuum of helping strategies for use when working with young mothers to ensure they have the necessary knowledge and skills to care effectively for their child.

Listening → Supporting → Teaching → Informing → Advising → Taking
direct action

How are we trying to empower the young mother to be an effective carer for her child? If we really want her to manage well, we need to start at the listening end of the continuum. If we fail at this point, she is unlikely to act on any useful advice and opportunities for learning we may offer. Once she is listened to and feels that we understand at least something of the way she sees her life, she will be more likely to allow us to help her. Doing things for her, taking direct action will help her little. It is important for *her* to be responsible and take charge, since she may have spent most of her life up to this point feeling controlled by others, not herself in charge of much. Indeed, one of the reasons behind her intended or actual parenthood may be a statement to the world that she is now making her own decisions. On the other hand, it is perhaps worth noting here that many young mothers did not plan to conceive and may not have wanted to; many may have endured pregnancy by default, as well as their subsequent motherhood. This is not to say that a mother in this situation does not want and love her baby; it is simply to remind us that motherhood in very young women may not always be the welcome state that most older mothers enjoy.

Any learning opportunities we provide have to be experiential for the mother so that she learns to do what is required on her own with confidence. Let me give an example.

A 15-year-old mother of a 13 month old is busy chatting with a friend while her daughter is crawling around, her fingers exploring everywhere. When she finds the electric sockets, her mother remains where she is and shouts at her to leave them alone and 'come back over here'. When the child stays exploring where she is, her mother goes over and grabs her, angrily telling her off, dragging her kicking and screaming back to where her friend is. She continues her conversation, while her daughter wanders off again.

How do we react to this? How do we help the mother to respond to her child in a more positive way? When a similar situation occurs, we can demonstrate how to do things differently; warn the child of the danger, of course, but there's no need to labour the point. Then divert the child's attention to something else of interest rather than telling her off and leaving it at that. We can demonstrate ways of speaking – gently, measured, warmly.

- Hey, look what I can see over here . . .
- Let's leave that; come with me and look at this . . .
- How about having a go with/a look at . . .
- Let's read a story together, play with . . .

The tone of voice is important, helping to normalise things. The young mother will see the benefits of responding to her child's behaviour in such a way almost immediately (contented child, unstressed mother) which should encourage her.

Play is an essential learning experience for children. However, some young mothers, who experienced difficult, abusive or neglectful childhoods, may not know how to play. They therefore do not know where to start with their own child. Play has to be demonstrated to the mother. I have seen many teenage mothers being quite rough in their play with their infants; also teasing in a bullying way. This sort of behaviour says a lot about how the mother was herself treated as a child and may well be treated still. It is no easy task to help her see that this is not what her child needs.

It needs to be explained – and demonstrated – that play is how children learn; that play is experiment, discovery, a means of self-expression and enjoyment. Play can be frustrating but it is a way for children to act out their feelings, experiences and fantasies. Play needs to happen for healthy, emotional development to occur as well as optimum physical growth and coordination. The best way to help young parents appreciate the importance of play is for the helper (whoever this is) to get down on the floor and play with their children. Reading too can be play. Very young mothers do not always appreciate that books have a place even in the life of a baby. Reading stories to children and singing to them are activities to which young parents may need to be introduced.

HANDLING OBSTRUCTIVE BEHAVIOUR

What is really difficult for a young mother – and father – is the fact that, although they need to focus on the needs of their child, they have urgent needs of their own to be met. The majority of teenagers still have a long way to go in their ego development; thus it is the hardest thing to let their own needs go and concentrate on another's. This is illustrated in the above example when the child of the young mother required her full attention and she needed to leave chatting to her friend until later. It is hard to defer gratification when young. Perhaps few of us are ready to do so until we reach at least our late teens; then it's a balancing act between seeing that our own needs are met and making sure those of our child are also.

It is generally a mistake to take at face value the confidence which the teenage mother endeavours to present to us. She may dismiss our proffered help not because she is self-reliant but because she is feeling unconfident, inadequate and fearful of letting this show. Her stress may manifest itself in anger, obstructiveness and rebellion or simply by her shutting down. Under such circumstances, no further learning is likely to take place. To avoid this happening, we must ensure that our communication is sensitive, clear and consistent. This will help her to respond in a similar way with her own child, learning to remain open, loving and calm however cross and difficult he becomes. The child then learns that his rages can be managed by his mother and that she is always completely 'there' for him.

GIVING CONSTRUCTIVE FEEDBACK

When working with a young mother, it is vital to offer her feedback on her mothering skills in a constructive, non-judgemental manner. The following example illustrates this point.

> *A nine-month-old baby girl has just been weighed. Her weight has suddenly gone up. The nursery nurse and health visitor say in the same breath: 'Too heavy'. 'I wrote "fatty piggy" on her card once before', says the health visitor jokingly to the 15-year-old mother. The mother feels criticised and demeaned. 'What've I gotta do – starve her?!' Her sense of humiliation expresses itself in indignation and furious sulks. She ends by screaming and repeating 'Don't bother! I'll weigh her myself. I'll feed her on tins and stuff. It's not my fault!'* (personal observation)

It is clear that the professionals' language was punitive, in spite of the fact that they had handled the child with loving care. The mother understandably was upset and as a result could not take anything in after the obvious disapproval expressed. Indeed, she worked herself up into quite a frenzy. The adults lost considerable ground in their relationship with this young mother. They may have thought they were teasing her, but it was ill judged. The rule here would be the Feedback Sandwich.

- Start with praise.
- Then mention something which could be worked on.
- Then return to praise.

There is always something to praise in any mother and bad news is generally received better after good. Constructive feedback, focusing on behaviour rather than the individual, provides a model for the mother to adopt with her child.

In a public place, I recently observed and overheard the following.

> *A child spilled orange juice down his front. The mother shouted: 'You stupid child! What a waste!'*

The young mother was furious. The incident caused her embarrassment and the child needed his clothes changed. Had she responded with, 'Never mind. Let's mop this mess up and put your cup somewhere where it won't get knocked over again', the child would have learned to be more careful and his self-esteem would have remained intact.

We have to model caring behaviour. A demonstration of touching and holding might help. What messages are being sent and received by the child, when the child is grabbed, plonked, shoved, squeezed, rushed as opposed to cuddled, snuggled, held comfortably and close? A baby knows how a parent is really feeling by her touch, her tone of voice and her eyes, whatever words are being said. This is necessary information for young parents to take on board.

We also need to demonstrate consistency and help the mother lay down positive rules for her child. Young parents find this particularly difficult, since many of them have not experienced consistent discipline themselves as children. Positive discipline provides emotional nourishment because it represents fixed norms and security.

INFANT FEEDING

Encouraging a young mother to breastfeed her baby and persevere through the difficult times can be a time-consuming task. She will reject breastfeeding in favour of the bottle for many reasons: breastfeeding hurts; she hasn't enough milk; her boyfriend doesn't like it; she doesn't want to expose her breasts. In the majority of cases, her reluctance comes down to one major factor – embarrassment. She doesn't like her baby 'nibbling at me like a little animal' (Hudson & Ineichen 1991). Many young mothers are confused about their body and their sexuality. Their sexual relationships may not have been very fulfilling or enlightening; they may not be very familiar with their body and not at all comfortable with it yet. Although it is frequently assumed that young mothers have nothing more to learn about sex, this is blatantly not the case. Helping a new, confused, shy young mother, whose emotions may be operating at a naïve level, to understand the benefits of breastfeeding and carry it out successfully require good communication skills, time and patience. It is also vital for us to be entirely at ease with our own bodies and with breastfeeding, if we are to help her be at ease with her body.

Young mothers (like older ones) may feel competitive about their child's development. Mixing a feed with an extra spoonful of formula is seen as beneficial to the baby's growth. Explanations need to be given clearly but without being patronising. If the mother feels attacked, she will not be able to take in what is being said to her.

CONCLUSION

Very young parents are often very frightened and it is not easy to empower them to be good-enough parents for their children. The challenges facing them range from managing their finances and relationships to continuing their emotional development and education, while learning how to be there for their child.

It is a great deal to ask. We can't achieve anything by scolding young parents, like the midwife who said to a group of schoolgirl mothers at their antenatal class: 'Why do you smoke? You shouldn't smoke! And you really mustn't wear shoes like that. They're very bad for your posture, you know . . .' (personal observation). We need to demonstrate emotional calm and unconditional regard for the young parent so that she can provide these for her child. The process of educating her in the care of her baby starts with attending to *her* needs and building up *her* emotional strength. It is important to encourage her to seek out further support from individuals and groups where she can find solidarity, mutuality and friendship.

If young parents are secure, confident and experiencing love themselves, there's a chance that they can commit themselves to the unselfish care of their child. They must take the responsibility for their learning and we are in a privileged position to provide some of those learning opportunities.

KEY POINTS

- Adolescents often find it difficult to accept advice; they do not want to be told what they should do.
- The majority of teenagers have a long way to go in their ego development; it is very hard for them to put their own needs to one side and concentrate on their child's.
- A young mother's world may lack the support she needs; she may not have had good models of fulfilling and loving relationships.
- The young mother is the expert on her experience to date.
- Once she has been listened to, she is more likely to allow herself to be helped.
- The principal task is to educate young parents in the importance of 'being there' for their children.

REFERENCES

Hadley E (ed) 1999 Tough choices: young women talk about pregnancy. The Women's Press, London

Hamlin M, Melling R, McMullen P, Vaughn M, Ward H 1998 Good for you. Nursery World, 8th January

Harris TA 1979 I'm OK – you're OK. Pan Books, London

Hudson F, Ineichen B 1991 Taking it lying down: sexuality and teenage motherhood. Macmillan Educational, London

Ingham R, Clements S, Stone N 2000 Teenage sexual knowledge, attitudes and behaviour in England: what is the relationship with deprivation? Centre for Sexual Health Research, University of Southampton

8 Education for adoptive parenting

Caroline Archer

INTRODUCTION

This chapter covers the following topics:
- the myth of trouble-free adoption
- impact of pre-, peri- and postnatal trauma on attachment and development
- psychobiological connections
- special needs of adoptive families
- developmental re-parenting: new beginnings
- sensory and emotional connections
- common presenting problems.

In the past, the special parenting needs of adopted children may have been obscured by society's desire for fairy-tale endings, where the 'untidy mess' of the single parent family (plus more recently the chaos of inadequate or abusive families) and the agony of childlessness could be resolved simply by removing the children involved and placing them in permanent, substitute families. Whilst few today would claim to hold to such simplistic beliefs, these 'happy ever after' myths are perpetuated not least by soap opera representations of adoptive family life and continue to influence society's perceptions of, and responses to, families created by adoption.

For many socially constructed families the lived experience may be very different as they struggle with the distressing, ongoing effects of their child's early traumatic experience. Research shows that adoptees are more likely than 'born-to' children to experience psychosocial problems, particularly conduct disorders, and to be referred to mental health services (Levy & Orlans 2000), whilst the incidence of specific learning difficulties, such as dyslexia, sensory integration difficulties, such as dyspraxia, and speech and language disorders is also raised in this population, even where the child has been placed in early infancy and without overt maltreatment (Archer 1999a).

CONSIDERATIONS FOR PARENTS ADOPTING BABIES AND YOUNG CHILDREN

One overwhelmingly powerful experience which is unique to adopted youngsters is abrupt severance of attachment to the birth mother. Since healthy attachments are the best protection against subsequent trauma (van der Kolk 1996), the adoptee is rendered particularly vulnerable to further stressors. The child may become sensitised to additional separations of even a transitory nature

(Archer 1999a, Levy & Orlans 2000, Verrier 1993) and may struggle with neurophysiological and neuropsychological sequelae which in adults could be termed post traumatic stress disorder (Hughes 2000). The youngster's trust in the safety of her world, the reliability of her caregivers and her knowledge of and belief in her self are often profoundly compromised. This is equally pertinent for babies relinquished at birth, since the infant's experience is of profound loss (Brodzinsky 1992) and abandonment (Verrier 1993) irrespective of adult motivations. As a consequence, the adopted infant remains in unregulated physiological arousal and may be difficult to comfort, often becoming hypervigilant, hyperreactive and resistant to subsequent nurture (Pickle 2000).

In many cases, the adopted infant's prebirth history is far from straightforward and the risks of subsequent developmental trauma far higher (Levy & Orlans 2000). Research has shown that significant events and emotions in the pregnant mother's life have a major impact on the developing fetus. Verny & Kelly (1982) provide evidence that extended periods of ambivalence about or rejection of the pregnancy can adversely affect fetal development; these emotions might be considered typical of many relinquishing birth mothers. Whilst the baby cannot be said to recognise the damaging affects to which he is exposed, he does experience them neurobiologically. Borysenko & Borysenko (1994) speak of a 'fetal–maternal dialogue', mediated by neurohormones and neuropeptides. For example, raised cortisol levels, demonstrable from 18 weeks gestation (Fisk 2000), form part of a pharmacological cascade in response to prolonged maternal distress. This can adversely affect the establishment of nerve pathways (Begley 1997) and the maturation of the hippocampal area of the midbrain, impeding the youngster's ability to regulate emotional arousal (Ladnier & Massanari 2000). A higher incidence of prematurity, low birth weight (Brazelton & Cramer 1991) and subsequent attentional deficits (Nachmias et al 1996) have also been associated with exposure to fetal stress hormones.

According to Schore (1994) the 'experience-dependent' maturation of the baby's brain and nervous system means that quite limited exposure to distressing emotional or sensory experiences during critical periods may have lasting developmental effects. This is particularly true of the first three years of life, including gestation, since 'neurons that fire together wire together' (Hebb 1949) and Perry (1999) has demonstrated that these are the years of exponential neural growth and differentiation. The initial plasticity is adaptive to survival, yet for the adoptee experiencing early trauma and then being placed in a healthier environment, it subsequently becomes maladaptive, when 'fight, flight and freeze' behaviours (Perry 1999) are 'hardwired' to expectations of further rejection or maltreatment (as neural networks are selectively burnt into the developing brain circuitry) and interfere with normal attachment processes (Archer 1999a, Hughes 1997). Again, the child's greatest source of resilience against further traumatic pathology, the primary attachment relationship between parent and infant, is likely to be seriously compromised (Hughes 2000). These early disturbances to the natural attachment process, in turn, can have lasting effects on the child's physical and cognitive as well as psychosocial development (Fahlberg 1994).

Youngsters of all ages placed for adoption may have been exposed to many highly significant risks in their formative months and years, which can compromise their attachment relationships and hence their physical and psychological health. Child abuse and neglect are obvious candidates here. More covert risks during the prenatal and perinatal period could include exposure to domestic violence, poor maternal nutrition or self-care, maternal abuse of drugs and alcohol, physical and emotional immaturity of the mother and birth complications (Pickle 2000). Children adopted from overseas are also likely to have faced overwhelming sensory distress and deprivation (Archer 1999a), whilst relinquished children with additional disabilities have frequently been subjected to batteries of clinical investigations, in order to establish the precise nature of their difficulties, and may have remained in the limbo of hospital or temporary foster homes for extended periods, due to the nature of their special needs or to uncertainties about their future. These circumstances pose additional risks of traumatisation to adoptees, compromising their already fragile sense of security and trust in the world (Levy & Orlans 1998, Pickle 2000).

In both prenatal and postnatal periods, the status of parental mental health is often highly relevant, in terms of both genetic and environmental factors (Siegel 1999). Factors in parents which may adversely affect the attachment and development of the child include chronic anxiety, often related to issues of poverty and social exclusion (Levy & Orlans 1998), lack of support through pregnancy or during the birth, ongoing maternal isolation, parents' own early attachment experiences, significant recent losses in the birth family, and clinical depressive states, personality disorders and psychosis (Levy & Orlans 1998, Schore 1994). The transmission of dysfunctional relationship patterns within families is a very significant factor in childhood abuse and neglect and may be particularly damaging to the child's development. It is vital to remember that the children at greatest risk of maltreatment, and hence those who are most likely to be placed for adoption eventually, may come from these most socially excluded families and those parents suffering the greatest mental distress themselves. However, in my experience, few adoptive parents will have been adequately prepared for the lasting social and behavioural difficulties they encounter in their children as a consequence of emotional distress in their birth families.

BOX 8.1	*Factors affecting the early development of babies and young children*

- Ambivalence about or rejection of pregnancy by parent(s)
- Highly charged events or emotions in parents' life
- Extended periods of parental distress – physical or emotional
- Parental abuse: drug-related or domestic violence
- Poor parental nutrition and healthcare
- Parental immaturity or lack of support
- Familial poverty and social exclusion
- Parents' personal attachment experiences
- Parental mental health difficulties
- Death of someone close to parents/child
- Child abuse, deprivation, neglect
- Separation(s) from birth mother (including for medical interventions)
- Child's health status and genetic factors

THE EDUCATIVE ROLE OF PRIMARY HEALTH PRACTITIONERS

By now it should be clear to readers that the early histories of adopted youngsters leave them with very special health and social care needs and their adoptive parents with equally special 'education for parenting' needs. Parenting an adopted child should not be considered the same as parenting a child born to the family (Archer 1999a). Mainstream parent education programmes such as SureStart and PIPPIN, which have been shown to be highly relevant to birth families (see elsewhere in this volume), may consequently be of less value to adoptive families. Since their experiences of parenting children may differ radically from those of friends and members of their family, adoptive parents will benefit from meeting others in similar circumstances, with whom they may share many of their natural anxieties, strengthen their self-confidence and increase their efficacy as parents (Archer 1999b, Moss 1997, Swanton & Arches 2000). Healthcare professionals should explore local, adoption-focused resources for adoptive families, in addition to making information and advice available to them, on an individual level, which acknowledge adoption and trauma-related issues.

EDUCATING AND SUPPORTING INFANT ADOPTERS

Awareness of these issues on the part of health practitioners can enable them to provide reassurance, information and advice to anxious adoptive parents in the early months post placement. Given their small numbers and geographical distribution, education for infant adopters at this stage is likely to remain on an individual level. Since most baby adopters will not have had opportunities to attend mainstream antenatal classes and will obviously not have had the standard nine months' physical and psychological preparation for parenthood, it is likely that these parents will feel particularly isolated and vulnerable. Parents' initial expectations of themselves may be high, having received their adoption agency's 'seal of approval', yet their assessment and preparation process is unlikely to have included a detailed discussion of infant development and the impact of early disrupted attachments. Hence adopters may require additional sensitive support and individually tailored parent education to come to terms with the challenges which 'instant' parenthood brings to their lives.

Initially, infant adopters will benefit from being encouraged to treat their infant as they would a premature or newborn baby, whether he is 10 days, 10 weeks or 10 months old on placement, in order to enhance developmental attachment processes (Archer 2000, Kupecky 1998). Parents should be made aware that even small changes to their baby's care and routine could trigger the release of stress hormones (Levy & Orlans 1998), leading to ongoing distress in the infant. Consistent, sensitive and informed handling from 'primary caregivers' is essential if the baby's distress is to be minimised and his fragile developmental trajectory repaired. This may mean that adopters would need to limit visits from family and friends in the early days, to allow the essential, biologically programmed bonding and attachment sequence (Hughes 1997, Siegel 1999) to become reestablished. Focus should be on establishing 'primary intersubjectivity', that wonderfully natural, two-way communication between parent and baby which we would hope to see begining at birth, before wider socioemotional relationships are encouraged. Through this developmental process the vulnerable infant can acquire the physiological and emotional co-regulation which is an essential precursor to mature self-regulation (Archer 2000).

Although health professionals will naturally be concerned for the infant's clinical needs and feeding and cleanliness routines in the early days, the emphasis for parents should be on establishing quiet 'rooming in' space, where the comfort, cuddles, playfulness and explorative, reciprocal interactions which form the essential early attachment communications between mother and infant can take place (Hughes 1997, Schore 1994). In addition, new parents should be made aware of their infant's potential hypersensitivity to sensory stimuli. Thus dim lights, softened sounds, familiar smells, gentle touch and movement are recommended (Levy & Orlans 1998). Where clinic or hospital visits or admissions are necessary, adopters should be particularly careful to minimise the environmental impact on their baby, by providing the reassurance of familiar faces, touch, sounds, smells and body movement (such as rocking) and through remaining with their youngster at all times. In these ways many of the baby's early feeding, sleeping and relationship difficulties can be reduced. This could be of particular relevance to adopters of youngsters with additional disabilities, who are more likely to require ongoing specialist interventions. It would benefit these parents greatly to understand that putting their children's attachment needs first will maximise their ultimate potential in all areas of learning and development.

BOX 8.2	*Educating and supporting adopters of infants*

- Provide reassurance and adoption-specific information.
- Help parents to understand that attachment is a two-way dialogue.
- Dispel notions that 'time and love' will be enough.
- Encourage parents to 'hear' and relate to their child in sensitive ways.
- Focus on enriching the child's sensory experience.
- Assist parents to 'network' with other adoptive families.
- Nurture the nurturers.

EDUCATING AND SUPPORTING ADOPTERS OF OLDER CHILDREN

It is vital that health practitioners dispel popular assumptions that time and love alone (Swanton & Archer 2000) can eradicate the trauma of the child's early years and avoid generalising from personal family and professional experiences of behavioural issues to reported difficulties in adoptive families. Frequently there are qualitative and quantitative differences between the behaviours of children in socially constructed and non-reconstituted families (Archer 1999b, Levy

& Orlans 1998). As we have seen, these have their basis in early neurobiological alterations and are reinforced by 'hardwired' distortions in the child's perceptions, expectations and behavioural responses, as they become organically etched into the child's brain circuitry. Failure to acknowledge these differences, attempting to provide reassurance with comments such as 'but all children do that' or assuming that family difficulties reflect fundamental parental dysfunction can lead to unnecessary alienation of the family seeking help (Archer 2000). This can exaggerate adopters' feelings of inappropriate self-blame, helplessness and isolation, make their invaluable task of re-parenting the child more arduous and increase the likelihood of placement disruption, with devastating outcomes for both child and family.

Unfortunately, few adoption agencies have yet reached the position of being able to provide this much-needed educational role to families prior to placement and post-placement support remains patchy. Furthermore, until a child has been placed with an individual family, it is often difficult to convey the extent of the emotional and physical challenge which parents may face (Archer 2000, Swanton & Archer 2000). Primary health professionals thus form part of a currently fragmented but essential post-placement support service, both through individual support work with adoptive families and alongside other childcare professionals, as part of the wider support network. They should be prepared to explore possibilities for creative interagency collaboration, both with statutory services and with voluntary bodies such as Adoption UK, who have played a pioneering role in the development of parent support programmes specifically for adoptive parents (see Resources at end of chapter).

Health practitioners seeking to provide parenting education directly to adopters should see their role primarily as supportive: nurturing the parents' strengths as the principal agents of therapeutic change (Kupecky 1998). They should aim to provide a non-judgemental sounding board for distressed parents, giving them space to explore the often contradictory emotions they experience. Understanding that these are frequently direct reflections of the conflicts and muddles besetting their child (Archer 1999b), and validating the good job parents are doing in picking up these difficult feelings are essential steps in this process (Archer 2000). This can lead directly to a focus on the reciprocal, non-verbal communications typical of very early attachment relationships (Schore 1994), for it is here that fundamental interruptions to development frequently occur and hence where healing can best be effected. Many traumatised children have received insufficient opportunities to develop their capacities for recognising and interpreting internal and external sensory experience at this stage. They therefore lack vital self-awareness (Schore 1994) in such basic areas as knowing when they are hungry and how to satisfy that need in appropriate ways. In this case binge eating, hoarding, excessive 'pickiness' or food refusal often result.

Helping adoptive parents explore playful and appropriate ways of providing additional opportunities for all forms of sensory and motor experience for their children, irrespective of chronological age, is essential to the development of sensory literacy and the enhancement of their overall well-being. For example, for a five year old who has spent much of her first years restricted to her cot, games to increase movement, body awareness, touch and eye contact could be appropriate. Parents might be encouraged to set aside regular times to hold their child on their knee in a rocking chair, whilst singing quietly or stroking her face or hair. They might also introduce nursery games, such as peek-a-boo, to establish object (parent) constancy, with plenty of additional tickles, giggles and fun to provide pleasurable touch and playful proximity experiences. Water play and splashing bath times might also be appropriate. However, all children are individuals and it is always the parent who is the expert on her child (Kupecky 1998). Health practitioners should therefore explore ways of drawing on parents' own strengths and intuition, when attempting to address a particular issue, working towards enhancing attachments within the family rather than intervening directly themselves.

Affective literacy, the ability to recognise, make sense of and manage emotions, is also frequently compromised in children who have experienced early separation, loss or maltreatment (Levy & Orlans 1998). Once again, it is through repeated 'good-enough' interactions in the developing attachment relationship between parent and infant that the child acquires the capacity to recognise both physical and psychological cues to his feelings, to name them and to regulate them appropriately (Archer 1999b, Schore 1994, Siegel 1999). Where early attachments have been compromised or the child exposed to the overwhelming trauma of maltreatment, poor emotional literacy and a weakened capacity to modulate emotional states at the nervous system level result. It then becomes vital that adoptive parents are provided with specific strategies to repair these affective deficits. Hence 'dealing with feelings' should form a major part of developmental re-parenting (Archer 1999b). Parents could be encouraged to exaggerate their own facial expressions, which have been shown to be central in the communication of emotion (Schore 1994, Siegel 1999) and to use their 'gut feelings' to tune into their child's emotions, so that they may verbalise, interpret and model regulation of basic affect states for her. Parents will in this way be utilising their own emotional awareness to provide additional learning opportunities for their troubled children.

EDUCATING AND SUPPORTING PARENTS ADOPTING CHILDREN FROM OVERSEAS

Children adopted from overseas frequently bring particular health issues with them. Johnson (1996) suggests that children arriving from developing countries should be screened routinely for intestinal parasites, nutritional deficiencies, HIV, sexually transmitted diseases, tuberculosis and hepatitis B and C, as well as for the early developmental and neurological disorders, such as auditory processing and coordination difficulties, which may be found in 'home-grown' maltreated children. Federici (1998) found a raised incidence of 'autistic-like' behaviours in this population, as the result of profound early sensory, motor and emotional deprivation. Since Baron-Cohen (1995) contends that autism is associated with abnormalities in the right orbitofrontal cortex, Federici's reports (1998) are consistent with Schore's findings (1994) that lack of appropriate early nurture can lead to functional deficits in this vital cortical area. Such children would also benefit from a sensori-emotional, developmentally based parenting programme to promote healthy attachments (Archer 1999a, 2000, Federici 1998).

The primary role of health professionals will be in providing information and sensitive support which promote this natural healing process and in helping adopters identify and meet other adoptive families locally. If all adoptive parents are routinely provided with information which allows them to begin re-laying the foundation stones of self-development through sensory, motor and emotional components, they can facilitate the development of newer, healthier neural connections (Archer 1999b, Perry 1999, Schore 1994) and a greater integration of self-awareness in their children. They will simultaneously begin damping down the maladaptive 'fight, flight and freeze' responses which are typical of traumatised children (Archer 1999b,c, Perry 1999), a pattern which is frequently gender related, with more boys tending to 'act out', via sympathetic nervous system dominance, and more girls 'acting in', through increased parasympathetic activity (Perry 1999, Schore 1994). It is primarily within the intimacy and safety of the parent–child relationship and through developmental re-parenting (Archer 1999c) that healthy alterations to the child's 'hard-wired' responses can eventually be brought about (Hughes 1997, Putnam 1997, Schore 1994).

COMMON PRESENTING PROBLEMS

Typically, adoptive parents of preschoolers will approach health professionals about difficulties such as tantrums, sleep problems, overactivity, eating, elimination, control and relationship issues. By the time they seek advice, they will often have tried most of the 'usual' management strategies with little success; the intensity, frequency and duration of these behaviours may well be challenging their belief in themselves as appropriate parents for their child.

It is essential that health practitioners acknowledge to parents the degree of difficulty they are facing, before helping them to explore the underlying trauma biology which underpins many of these issues. A traumatised youngster may be unable to settle for sleep or be wakeful during the night because being in her bedroom repeatedly reminds her of the terror of being left alone, or sexually abused, in her birth family (Archer 1999b). Similarly, youngsters will often express their distress through the physical and verbal opposition typical of tantrums, through raised levels of activity or lethargy, by becoming intensely clingy or seeking attention indiscriminately. By helping parents distinguish between age and stage-appropriate and inappropriate behaviours and providing them with insights into the aetiology of the difficulties, they will then be more able to care for their child effectively. For example, providing containment for the child's outburst during a tantrum, by remaining with the child and holding him gently, whilst speaking quietly and empathically of possible reasons for his distress may be far more effective than ignoring the behaviour in the hope that it will abate. In addition, reframing the child's problems as attempts to resolve underlying difficulties (Swanton & Archer 2000) can increase parents' ability to respond calmly under stress and avoid unwitting retraumatisation of their child.

More generally, health professionals may need to redirect adopters' very natural desire to 'bring on' a child who may be lagging behind developmentally or to measure him against normal developmental milestones. Enthusiasm should be tempered by an exploration of the adopted child's history of attachment breaks and maltreatment and a realistic acknowledgement of the impact these will have on the child's physical and cognitive as well as psychosocial development, since unresolved attachment disturbances have been shown adversely to affect intellectual and physical (Fahlberg 1994) as well as social, emotional and spiritual development (Archer 1999a, Levy & Orlans 1998, 2000). Hence, encouraging parents to be sensitive to the youngster's need to go at his own pace, perhaps permitting him to regress to earlier stages which were interrupted by separation, loss and distress, could relieve parents' anxieties and provide them with more developmentally appropriate intervention strategies, to the ultimate benefit of their child (Archer 1999c). Whilst providing stimulation for a child is an essential component of healthy development, the child's overriding needs are to be helped to recover from early traumatic experience and to be accepted for who and what he is right now. Assisting parents to understand that working on attachment and early developmental issues forms the basis for promoting global developmental maturity is an essential educative role for all health professionals.

As the adopted child becomes older, he may increasingly display aggressive or non-compliant behaviours, typical of conduct and oppositional defiant disorders, in addition to the impulsive and attentional difficulties associated with attention deficit disorders. Here again, healthcare workers should explore the trauma histories of youngsters with parents sensitively, so that they can recognise the underlying nature of their child's difficulties (Waters 1998). In this way they can assist parents not only in identifying the most appropriate forms of therapeutic intervention but also by providing them with a deeper understanding of their child. This may alleviate much of the guilt and confusion which can so easily impair adoptive parents' confidence at this point (Archer 2000).

Thus supported, parents will be more able to draw on their reserves of patience with the child, to explore ways of assisting him to recognise and avoid unnecessary traumatic triggers and to engage in strategies which directly regulate his arousal. Initially this should be through shared 'co-regulatory' activities between parent and child, such as taking time out together rather than expecting the child to calm down alone. This recapitulates the co-regulation experiences intrinsic to the good-enough (Winnicott 1965) parent–infant relationship. An understanding of the biological implications of secondary traumatisation (Cairns 1999) will also help practitioners to see beyond the obvious distress of parents themselves and enable them to provide a safe and empathic environment within which adopters can express their understandable fears and concerns about and for their child. Consequently parents will be much better placed to address their child's challenging behaviours with renewed vigour, confidence and humour and to become the 'steel box with the velvet lining' (Moss 1997) such children require.

SUMMARY

In short, the role of the health professional in relation to all adoptees is one of providing a 'holding environment' (Winnicott 1965) for child and family. Whilst initially this may involve some direct caregiving, it should wherever possible give way to 'nurturing the nurturer' and hence allowing the 'growth-promoting environment' (Schore 1994) of the adoptive family to flourish. Adopters come to the task of parenting with a wealth of commitment, energy and enthusiasm but have often been given little real preparation for adoptive family life. Health practitioners are therefore uniquely placed to provide invaluable educational opportunities for parents to explore the impact of their child's traumatic beginnings on her ongoing physical and psychological health. In strengthening their knowledge base and through non-judgemental counselling, practitioners can then draw on parents' natural strengths and insights and enable them to fulfil their role as the principal agents of healing for their children (Kupecky 1998).

KEY POINTS

- Adopted infants experience the 'primal wound' of separation.
- Early trauma leads to changes at the neurobiological level.
- Adopted children may think, feel and respond in unique ways.
- Adoptive parents are the major agents of healing for their children.
- These are committed parents undertaking a challenging task.
- There are essential differences between birth and adoptive parenting.
- The educative role of healthcare professionals will be predominantly at the individual level.
- Parents' distress frequently reflects their child's distress.
- Non-judgemental, active listening is essential.
- Help parents put the fun back into family life.
- Intervene sooner rather than later.
- Establish interdisciplinary working.
- Use an attachment-based developmental re-parenting programme.
- Adopters need reassurance from 'someone who really knows'.
- Further information, training and support for both professionals and adopters is available from Adoption UK (details below).

REFERENCES

Archer C 1999a First steps in parenting the child who hurts: tiddlers and toddlers. Jessica Kingsley, London

Archer C 1999b Next steps in parenting the child who hurts: tykes and teens. Jessica Kingsley, London

Archer C 1999c Re-parenting the traumatised child: a developmental process. Young Minds 42:42–43

Archer C 2000 Living with a child with severe emotional and behavioural difficulties. In: Making sense of attachment in adoptive and foster families. Adoption UK, Northamptonshire, pp 74–82

Baron-Cohen S 1995 Mindblindness: an essay on autism and theory of mind. MIT Press, Cambridge, Mass

Begley S 1997 How to build a baby's brain. Newsweek Spring/Summer: 28–32

Borysenko J, Borysenko M 1994 The power of the mind to heal. Hay House, Carson, California

Brazelton T, Cramer B 1991 The earliest relationship. Karnac Books, London

Brodzinsky D 1992 A stress and coping model of adoption adjustment. In: Brodzinsky D, Schechter M (eds) The psychology of adoption. Oxford University Press, New York, pp 3–24

Cairns K 1999 Surviving paedophilia. Trentham Books, Stoke-on-Trent

Fahlberg V 1994 A child's journey through placement. BAAF, London

Federici R 1998 Help for the hopeless child: a guide for families. Federici and Associates, Alexandria, Virginia

Fisk N 2000 Does a foetus feel pain? The Times 28 March

Hebb D 1949 The organization of behavior: a neurophysiological theory. John Wiley, New York

Hughes D 1997 Facilitating developmental attachment. Jason Aronson, Northvale, New Jersey

Hughes D 2000 Clinical editorial. Connections: Journal of the Association for Treatment and Training in the Attachment of Children August:2

Johnson D 1996 Presentation to PNPIC Conference, Cleveland, Ohio

Kupecky R 1998 Families: major channel for change and healing. Connections: Journal of the Association for Treatment and Training in the Attachment of Children August:5–6

Ladnier R, Massanari A 2000 Treating ADHD as attachment deficit hyperactivity disorder. In: Levy T, Orlans M (eds) Handbook of attachment interventions. Academic Press, New York, pp 27–63

Levy T, Orlans M 1998 Attachment, trauma and healing. Child Welfare League of America, Washington DC

Levy T, Orlans M 2000 Attachment disorder and the adoptive family. In: Levy T, Orlans M (eds) Handbook of attachment interventions. Academic Press, San Diego, pp 243–259

Moss K 1997 Integrating attachment theory into special needs adoption. Beech Brook, Cleveland, Ohio

Nachmias M, Gunnar M, Mangelsdorf S, Parritz R, Buss K 1996 Behavioral inhibition and stress reactivity: moderating role of attachment security. Child Development 67:508–522

Perry B 1999 The memories of states: how the brain stores and retrieves traumatic experience. In: Goodwin J, Attias R (eds) Splintered reflections: images of the body in trauma. Basic Books, New York, pp 9–38

Pickle P 2000 Community-focused attachment services. In: Levy T, Orlans M (eds) Handbook of attachment interventions. Academic Press, New York, pp 261–277

Putnam F 1997 Dissociation in children and adolescents, a developmental perspective. Guilford Press, New York

Schore A 1994 Affect regulation and the origin of the self. Lawrence Erlbaum, New Jersey

Siegel D 1999 The developing mind. Toward a neurobiology of interpersonal experience. Guilford Press, New York

Swanton P, Archer C 2000 Adoption: changes in the light of experience. In: White K (ed) The changing face of child care. NCVCCO, London, pp 167–179

van der Kolk B 1996 The complexity of adaptation to trauma. In: van der Kolk B, McFarlane A, Weisaeth L (eds) Traumatic stress: the effects of overwhelming experience on mind, body and society. Guilford Press, New York, pp 182–213

Verny T, Kelly J 1982 The secret life of the unborn child. Collins, Glasgow

Verrier N 1993 The primal wound. Gateway, Baltimore, Maryland

Waters F 1998 Parents as partners in the treatment of dissociative children. In: Silberg J (ed) The dissociative child. Diagnosis, treatment, and management, 2nd edn. Sidran Press, Lutherville, Maryland

Winnicott D 1965 The family and individual development. Tavistock, London

RESOURCES

The theoretical and practical bases for developmentally based parenting programmes are explored in greater detail in *First Steps in Parenting the Child Who Hurts: Tiddlers and Toddlers*, Caroline Archer, Jessica Kingsley, London, 1999, and *Next Steps in Parenting the Child Who Hurts: Tykes and Teens*, Caroline Archer, Jessica Kingsley, London, 1999. These books are available from high street booksellers or by mail order from: BAAF Publications, Skyline House, 200 Union Street, London SE1 0LX.
Tel: 0207 593 2001

The principles outlined in these books have directly informed the development of Adoption UK's Parent Support Programme, *It's a Piece of Cake?* For further information, contact: Adoption UK, Manor Farm, Appletree Road, Chipping Warden, Banbury, Oxfordshire OX17 ILH.
Helpline: 0870 7700 450
Admin: 01295 660121

9 Supporting parents with learning difficulties

Sue McGaw, Debbie Valentine and Alex Clark

INTRODUCTION

This chapter shares the good practice of the Special Parenting Service (SPS) which currently runs as a stand-alone arm of the Learning Disability Directorate of an NHS Trust in Cornwall. Over the past 13 years this pioneering service has enjoyed working with and supporting over 600 parents with learning disabilities, many of whom have presented with an array of simple and complex needs. The service has also conducted five research programmes, provided multi-agency training across the UK and developed theoretical models and practical resources to aid professional practice, for the purpose of providing a better service for families. To share some of the best and most useful aspects of our work with readers, this chapter will answer some of the most common questions put to us by professionals over the years.

- What are the needs of parents who have a learning disability?
- What issues need to be considered prior to the first interview?
- What issues need to be covered during an interview?
- How can parents be helped to explore their particular needs?
- How can we assess parents' abilities and their children's well-being?
- What type of support should we offer a parent who has a learning disability?
- What helps a teaching programme to be successful?
- What specific methods should we use?
- How will we know if our programme is successful?

Despite newspaper articles, surveys, studies and reports over the past 20 years that have drawn attention to the needs and plight of parents with disabilities and their children, there are few quality services available within the UK to provide advice, support and guidance to parents with learning disabilities. At last, the recently published National Strategy on Learning Disabilities (DoH 2001) and Jigsaw of Services Report (Goodinge 2000) give credence and legitimacy to professional concerns that they are untrained, underresourced and underfunded when it comes to supporting a parent who happens to have a learning disability. The dilemma is that despite this discrepancy, professionals are required to 'soldier on' and do their best.

WHAT ARE THE NEEDS OF PARENTS WHO HAVE A LEARNING DISABILITY?

This chapter focuses on the areas of parenting which parents with a learning disability are likely to find difficult and outlines how to approach and assess their needs, as well as their children's needs. In general, parents who have a learning disability tend to present with multiple needs which might range from difficulties with housing and finance to mental health issues or relationship problems. The most vulnerable areas for parents often include the following.

Children's development

Children of parents with learning disabilities, it has been suggested, are more vulnerable to delays in cognitive and expressive language domains (Feldman et al 1986, McGaw 1994). It has also been found that a child's language and per-ceptual-cognitive competence are strongly related to the amount of stimulation provided by the parent and that both are reliable indicators of developmental delay. Amongst the parents assessed by SPS, lowered rates of, for example, language and motor stimulation are frequent.

Neglect and abuse

Research has shown that purposeful abuse on the part of a learning-disabled mother is probably rare and that incidences of abuse are more commonly perpetrated by someone associated with the mother, e.g. partner/relative (Koller & Richardson 1988, Tymchuk & Andron 1990). It appears that, due to a lack of parental education and/or a paucity of social support, neglect of children's needs is a more prevalent cause of problems for children of parents with a learning disability. A high percentage of children of these parents are placed on Child Protection Registers.

Healthcare and safety

The few studies examining parental knowledge in conjunction with a learning disability suggest that a proportion of these parents have limited knowledge and few of the practical skills necessary for the adequate provision of healthcare and safety for their children (Tymchuk 1998, Tymchuk et al 1999). Of major concern is the fact that this lack of knowledge is most likely to become apparent in emergencies which require the highest levels of understanding in order to identify and understand the importance of symptoms and respond appropriately. It is, of course, in these situations that a child will be at greatest risk of harm.

Parental factors

Parental inadequacy may be predicted if the parent has high levels of stress, a low IQ (below 60), poor academic skills (e.g. reading ability), poor cognitive skills (decision making, problem solving) and poor child interactional skills (e.g. non-empathic) (Tymchuk & Andron 1992). Additional risk factors affecting levels of parenting ability might include a history of childhood abuse, evidence of psychopathology and a negative maternal attitude towards parenting (Tymchuk & Andron 1992). Socioeconomic factors such as poverty, social isolation and presence or absence of family support, as well as environmental factors such as housing, heating, having a telephone, transport and access to amenities, can have considerable influence on parenting competence.

WHAT ISSUES NEED TO BE CONSIDERED PRIOR TO THE FIRST INTERVIEW?

Engaging parents

The point of engagement with a family will be critical to the way that the parents accept and receive help. Ultimately, parental cooperation with professionals is essential so that the right level of support can be arranged to suit the parents' needs. It is extremely beneficial to parents and their child that they are offered (and hopefully accept) help and support at an early stage of the child's development (McGaw 2000). One way to ensure that such engagement is successful is to arrange a joint initial visit with someone whom the family already trusts and who is aware of the parents' particular learning disabilities.

Timing

Parents are much more likely to benefit from appropriately timed involvement with services (McGaw 2000). Some forward planning and prioritisation of needs can help to avoid problems associated with the repetition of assessments and families feeling overwhelmed by a large number of professionals working in the home.

Honesty

Honesty is always the best policy with parents with learning disabilities, whatever the professional opinion and especially when it relates to a parent's competency. Parents will find it difficult to trust you if they are misled as to your perception of their parenting abilities and you appear to have two agendas. When there are concerns, the SPS always discusses these frankly with parents first, before sharing these concerns with other people.

Labelling

Some parents take offence at being called 'learning disabled' and do not accept this diagnosis regardless of professional criteria. Other parents prefer different terms which describe their particular learning disability. Whatever the preferred terminology, getting it right will prove vital to maintaining a positive and productive relationship with that particular parent.

Tact and sensitivity

Both of these are essential when tackling issues of disability. Related stigmatisation and fears about the intentions of professionals may, perhaps, be produced by continual involvement with services.

WHAT ISSUES NEED TO BE COVERED DURING AN INTERVIEW?

Questions parents commonly ask

Why are you here?

Stressing that the purpose of your involvement is to give *positive* advice and support should help to allay the fears of parents who may be concerned about their child's removal.

What are you going to do?

Giving a clear and detailed explanation, with pictorial handouts/leaflets (with a low readability level – approximate reading level of the *Sun* newspaper) will allow parents to get an idea of your intentions and will also help you to foster a trusting relationship with the family.

Can you get me a new house?

Parents might have unrealistic expectations of your influence over other services. You will need to explain clearly what you can and cannot provide in terms of information, guidance, teaching, advocacy and resources. Parents often get confused as to which organisation you represent, what your role is and the powers you have within it. The penalty of not clarifying this is ejection from the household because you did not 'come up with the goods'.

Never mind that, are you going to help me get them to bed?

You may be required to repeat and clarify your overall programme of support and its aims and objectives, if a parent's expectation about your role is inaccurate or unrealistic.

How many times do I have to tell them? Why won't they listen to me?

Parents who express their difficulties with behaviour management in terms of their 'problem child' will require some sensitive prompting to initiate changes in their own behaviour. Deliberating about the pros and cons of behavioural management is not always the most direct route to create change with parents who experience difficulties with abstract concepts. Simply showing the parents how to respond to a situation by asking them to copy what you do is a good starting point. Video the situation if you can. Parents will recognise the positive changes in their child and themselves over time, especially if you use video feedback.

Definitely the wrong things to say to parents

I am going to carry out an intelligence test to help me to assess your parenting

Parents can become very confused and anxious about the implications of an intelligence test or any other test. It is much easier for all concerned if an assessment is described in terms of understanding which areas of parenting they find more or less difficult. Let them know that you recognise that all parents are different in the way that they learn about parenting and the skills that they bring to this job.

I promise that I won't let Social Services take your children away

During the initial visit, explain in simple language that you are legally obliged to communicate with other professionals about child protection issues that might materialise during your involvement with the family. *It is vital that you are always careful about the legal aspects of Child Protection and are aware of the protocols laid down by your local Area Child Protection Committee.*

What you need to do is...

In order to build up a positive, respectful relationship with parents, ensure that they are given choices and opportunities which promote autonomy and control over their children's lives. Whilst professionals should tactfully guide, rather than instruct parents, a fine balance needs to be achieved between giving clear, distinct directions and subtle prompting. Consequently, much depends upon the parents' level of understanding and the circumstances.

HOW CAN PARENTS BE HELPED TO EXPLORE THEIR PARTICULAR NEEDS?

During an initial visit, it may seem a daunting prospect to be responsible for providing support to people with such complex needs. However, it will be beneficial to establish early on what it is that parents are hoping to gain from your efforts. Always ask them, rather than make assumptions about their needs. Giving positive acknowledgement to parents regarding their strengths and explaining what is needed in terms of 'areas requiring a bit more help or support' may help them to relax.

Joan was referred following the birth of her sixth child. On visiting the home, it was discovered that the family were living in cramped conditions with just two bedrooms. Joan's husband was providing practical support but little emotional input and he was drinking heavily. One of the children had recently been excluded from school following displays of extremely challenging behaviour. All six children appeared on the Child Protection Register. Joan's health was suffering as a result. She was known to have a learning disability, having attended a Special Educational School throughout her teenage years.

Here, the natural service response would be to establish the most vital areas of care and support which might be offered to parents with learning disabilities. However, whilst services can be keen to engage parents such as Joan and her husband, the couple are anxious about discussing their difficulties with strangers and exposing any 'weaknesses' in their parenting. The SPS approach is as follows.

- Provide parents with a calling card with our name, title, agency address and telephone number to let them know who we are.
- Ensure that we convey respect, warmth, empathy and understanding when talking and listening to parents' experiences, their anxieties and concerns.
- Simplify our language. If in doubt, we ask parents if they understand the meaning of what we have said and audio-tape the conversation for the parent to play back at leisure, if the content is detailed.
- Check parents' reading, writing, numerical and time-telling abilities, before asking them to complete forms or questionnaires. We explain that we work with many parents who have difficulties with reading, writing, sums, using clocks, etc. and check whether they find this difficult as well.
- Use a checklist such as the 'I Need Help . . . ' (see Parent Assessment Manual, Box 9.1) to establish strengths and weaknesses across parenting and child domains. When using a five-point Likert Scale, we start at the extreme ends, e.g. 'Are you coping and don't need help?', 'Are you not coping at all?' or 'Are you some place in the middle?'.
- Ask parents what they want and need, in terms of resources, support, teaching, etc. We help parents to prioritise areas or skills for teaching by drawing different size boxes and ask parents to point to the box depicting the 'size' of their need.
- Give plenty of choices with regard to the type of support which is offered. This can help to instil a feeling of empowerment in parents who have learning disabilities. The sense that a parent is helping him/herself rather than purely receiving help from others is very important.
- Achieve a balance between giving too much choice (which can often result in confusion and a sense of being overwhelmed by multiple factors) and not providing enough choices.

HOW CAN WE ASSESS PARENTS' ABILITIES AND THEIR CHILDREN'S WELL-BEING?

Assessing parenting is in itself a complicated and highly subjective process. Inevitably, when parents appear to be coping with their parenting and their children are thriving and developing appropriately, there is no need for an assessment of their caretaking abilities. Conversely, when a child's health, safety, development or general well-being is jeopardised in some way, statutory agencies are obliged to scrutinise the quality of the parenting to see if this, along with a number of other factors, is responsible for the child's condition. However, when this situation involves a parent with a learning disability, professionals need to be aware of pejorative attitudes and assumptions which might prejudge parental competencies, currently or in the future. It is therefore important to establish whether the quality and frequency of parenting practices are the negative components affecting the child's care and development or whether other extraneous factors are responsible (McGaw & Sturmey 1994).

At present, there are very few assessments designed specifically for use with parents with learning disabilities. However, the Framework for the Assessment of Children in Need and their Families (DoH 2000) and accompanying training pack The Child's World (Horwath 2000) now offer some suggestions for assessing parents who have a learning disability. Within this document, the Parent Assessment Manual (PAM) (McGaw et al 1998), produced by SPS, is recommended for the purpose of establishing what parents might need to learn.

Drawing on the Parental Skills Model (McGaw & Sturmey 1994), the PAM was designed to assess three main indicators of adequate parenting. The child's care and development (a primary indicator of adequate parenting) is influenced by (a) the parent's life skills, (b) the family history and (c) the support and resources available to the parent (otherwise known as secondary indicators).

BOX 9.1	*The Parent Assessment Manual*

The Parent Assessment Manual is a holistic functional assessment package which provides a comprehensive overview of the learning-disabled parent's abilities with respect to various parenting domains.

- The PAM assesses vital aspects of childcare across 10 domains including feeding, healthcare, hygiene, warmth and stimulation of the child's development.
- The parent's life skills are measured across 24 domains in terms of their functional abilities (e.g. time telling, budgeting) and parenting skills, such as promoting safety and establishing household routines.
- The level of support and resources available to a parent from his/her family, friends or the local community is also examined.
- A detailed family history allows the professional to assess whether the parent has any experience of appropriate childrearing models.
- A strengths and needs risk profile can be put together in a visual form to help professionals prioritise a teaching programme and service involvement.
- The PAM also provides a comparison of professionals' and parents' perceptions of their needs.
- Throughout the PAM, the format has been modified to suit people with learning disabilities using simplified text and illustrations to enhance understanding of the tasks and scenarios.

Also, the PAM was developed using a contingency model (McGaw 1998) which links parenting knowledge to parenting skills and practice. Research has shown that teaching parents by imparting knowledge may not result in improvements in skills (Bakken et al 1993). For this reason, the PAM assesses parents' knowledge *and* skills, whilst also measuring whether the parents practise their skills with adequate frequency.

Other functional assessments

In the absence of standardised measures for use with parents with learning disabilities, functional assessments examining more specific domains of functioning have been developed.

HOME: Home Observation for Measurement of the Environment (Caldwell & Bradley 1984)

The HOME looks at the responsiveness of the parent and levels of stimulation within the home environment. It also looks into the disciplinary restrictions placed on the child. The test comprises a checklist covering areas of parental behaviour including:

- emotional and verbal responsivity
- acceptance of child's behaviour
- organisation of environment
- provision of play materials.

There are three checklists available, corresponding to different child age groups. The test is a good way of establishing how the parent and child interact within the home environment.

Home Inventory of Dangers and Safety Precautions 2 (Tymchuk et al 1999)

This tool, designed for health, education and disability-based professionals, will help to identify hazards and precautions present in the home such that injuries and accidents can be prevented. The assessment is a comprehensive checklist covering, for example, fire, electrical and poison-related hazards. A good measure of health and safety issues.

Ohio Functional Assessment Battery (Olsson 1994)

This selection of tools contains both full length and quick tests of functional living skills. The comprehensive version enables the professional to measure performance on a series of everyday practical skills including money management, organisation of time and following directions. In addition, the Functional Living Skills Assessment covers self esteem, nonverbal communication and decision making. A good overall assessment of practical abilities.

First Steps to Parenthood (Young & Strouthos 1997)

This assessment contains simple questions for the parent at various stages of pregnancy and motherhood as the child develops. Each set of questions is accompanied by an illustration. The aim is to initiate discussion of the salient issues of parenting. A more accessible tool to use with parents with learning disabilities.

Psychometric and developmental assessment

Psychometric assessments of intellectual functioning (e.g. WAIS: Wechsler 1988) can be administered by a psychologist. A referral may be the best way to ensure that the parents' level of intellectual functioning is properly documented and interpreted. This information is vital for implementing a teaching programme which will be understood by the parent.

A full developmental assessment might also be useful in measuring developmental delays in the children of parents with learning disabilities. Such information could be very useful in attempting to improve stimulation to specific areas of a child's functioning. Assessments such as the Griffiths Mental Development Scales (in Huntley 1996), the Bayley Infant Scales 2 (Bayley 1993) and the Schedule of Growing Skills (Bellman et al 1996) should be used by someone who is knowledgeable about their properties and trained in their administration, e.g. clinical psychologist, health visitor, paediatrician.

Key messages

- Parents with learning disabilities commonly present with a wide range of strengths and difficulties that should be viewed within the context of an 'overall picture'. Areas of vulnerability should be discreetly assessed using a systematic approach which takes into account the well-being of the child (their care and development) in relation to the parents' individual, and combined, parental competencies.
- Relevant issues to consider before an initial visit might include how to engage the parent through the use of tact and honesty. We need to be sensitive to the use of 'labels', especially as parents usually prefer to see themselves as a 'mum or dad' to their child, not as a parent with a learning disability.
- During an interview, parents with learning disabilities often become confused about which agency you represent and why you are there. Be prepared with simple, written information (perhaps with a photograph of yourself), with a contact number and encourage parents to call your agency, to check out your credentials.
- Providing praise, remaining non-judgemental and conveying warmth and understanding to the parents are essential parts of forming a relationship. Asking the parents about their needs and offering sufficient choices can help professionals to provide useful and appreciated levels of support.
- Despite the paucity of assessments that can be used with parents with learning disabilities, the Parent Assessment Manual provides a comprehensive overview of a parent's abilities using a format which is accessible to this population. The PAM deals with three major predictors of parenting performance and draws together information about a parent's knowledge, skills and practice.

WHAT TYPE OF SUPPORT SHOULD WE OFFER A PARENT WHO HAS A LEARNING DISABILITY?

Once the specific needs of the family have been identified, prioritised teaching programmes and appropriate levels of support can be developed. It has been identified that the most critical predictor of adequate parenting for people with learning disabilities is the frequency and quality of support provided to them (McGaw & Sturmey 1994). Programmes of support must be individually tailored to meet the needs of both parent and child and use specialised training strategies (McGaw 2000). There are many types of support required by parents with learning disabilities.

Support with parenting skills which relate to the primary and secondary needs of the child

These skills include health, safety, hygiene, child development, guidance and control, parental responsiveness and stimulation, all of which are critical to the development and well-being of the child.

Support with skills which help parents with learning disabilities to live independently in the community

Essential practical life skills which directly or indirectly affect parenting competencies include literacy, numeracy, time telling, budgeting, problem solving, decision making, home management, self-care and vocational development.

Often parents who need practical help and resources won't necessarily feel able or competent to access these for themselves and will be dependent upon services to acquire resources on their behalf such as transportation, respite care, housing, financial assistance, clothing, family planning and household needs.

Support with essential social skills

Social skills which affect parents' ability to acquire resources, manage relationships and feel good about themselves relate to verbal language, self-esteem, assertiveness and stress and anger management.

Providing advocacy to families is essential especially if they have limited social skills and difficulties expressing their wishes and opinions at core groups, case conferences, planning meetings and care proceedings.

Administering a holistic and comprehensive assessment to identify the specific needs of the child and parent will assist in identifying and prioritising the teaching programmes that require immediate intervention. The parenting assessments undertaken by the SPS incorporate the perception of the families' needs by an involved professional, the parents' understanding of their own needs and finally the knowledge, skills and practice assessed by the SPS.

WHAT HELPS A TEACHING PROGRAMME TO BE SUCCESSFUL?

Current research, although limited, indicates that the most successful teaching programmes are those that:

- use educators who are flexible, adaptable in their approach and sensitive in their manner. They should not be patronising and need to identify and build on the strengths of the family to promote engagement with services
- are paced and presented at an appropriate level for the parent (verbal comprehension, reading ability of approximately 6–13 years)
- focus on performance-based strategies rather than knowledge based, as parents face difficulties when attempting to generalise and maintain newly acquired knowledge and skills
- optimise learning and teach two or three programmes at any one time. However, when teaching new programmes, it will also be necessary to reinforce your past teaching (Bakken et al 1993)
- do not overwhelm parents by addressing too many skills at any one time; ideally, two home-based visits per week tapering off to one visit per week, for an approximate period of 3 months
- include an additional 3-month extension to help parents practise newly learnt skills so that they become overlearnt (thus ensuring maintenance and generalisation). It is important to continue to reinforce all taught programmes throughout the 6-month intervention and possibly for up to one year. The research substantiates that long-term, ongoing support is more beneficial to parents rather than short-term teaching.

A number of key concepts and principles have been identified as promoting learning and empowering parents such that they can develop their self-esteem, internal control, problem-solving skills, social interactions and comprehension of social roles (Espe-Sherwindt et al, 1990).

- Be both positive and proactive in interactions with families.
- Offer help in response to family-identified needs.
- Permit the family to decide whether to accept or reject help.
- Offer help that is normative.
- Offer help that is congruent with the family's appraisal of its needs.
- Promote acceptance of help by keeping the response costs low.
- Permit help to be reciprocated.
- Empower the family to achieve immediate success in mobilising resources.
- Promote the use of informal support as the principal way of meeting needs.
- Promote a sense of cooperation and joint responsibility for meeting family needs.
- Promote the family members' acquisition of effective behaviour for meeting needs.
- Promote the family members' ability to see themselves as responsible for their behaviour change.

WHAT SPECIFIC TEACHING METHODS SHOULD WE USE?

Step-by-step teaching instructions and visual aids are the preferred methods of teaching for parents with learning disabilities. Praise and reinforcement are crucial to stimulate parents' continuing efforts during the teaching programme. Both individual home-based teaching programmes and group intervention are methods espoused by the SPS and found to be the most successful in empowering parents to enhance family preservation.

Individual home-based teaching

Individually designed programmes which use behavioural techniques, e.g. cueing, prompting, modelling, reinforcement, forward and backward chaining, role play, need to be designed by professionals trained in these techniques.

The following is a case study of a current intervention being undertaken by the SPS. Immediate teaching was required in the areas of feeding, guidance and control, and supervision of children. The programme was provided for an initial 3-month period and extended to 6 months. It is envisaged that ongoing support and reinforcement of teaching will be provided by other professionals (family aide, Mencap, health professionals and family members).

CASE STUDY

The Special Parenting Service Intervention: the Smith family

Background

Mr Smith is a single parent fathering a 6-year-old daughter and 5-year-old son diagnosed with fragile X syndrome. The teaching programmes required had been identified by a psychologist using the Parent Assessment Manual, the guardian ad litem and social worker (Parent Skills Index). It was felt by SPS that due to severely challenging behaviour exhibited by the son, teaching on guidance and control (how to deal with tantrums) would be most beneficial so that Mr Smith could progress with teaching in the other two areas.

Specific skills

- Guidance and control: parent manages child's disruptive behaviour.
- Feeding: parent provides nutritious meals, drinks throughout the day and healthy snacks.
- Supervision: parent supervises children when outdoors.

Teaching methods

Teaching methods incorporated the use of ABC charts (antecedents, behaviours, consequences) to identify causes of anger, tantrums and parent's responses to the behaviour. Handouts on appropriate discipline techniques, positive communication skills, modelling, role play, visual prompts and video feedback were utilised. Following teaching on providing well-balanced meals and healthy snacks, a food diary was completed by the parent on a daily basis. Role play, descriptive scenarios and videos were used to provide teaching on child protection and safety outdoors (road safety, playing outdoors in inclement weather and protection from unsuitable individuals).

Results

Programme efficacy was measured by frequency observation charts (PAM) on all the above skills (completed by SPS and Social Services during each visit). The results were then charted and revealed that considerable improvement in all areas had been observed. In addition, the food diary also demonstrated increased feeding abilities.

Group interventions

Whilst individual programmes can be an extremely effective method of working with parents, the most powerful approach is one that combines intensive home-based teaching with group interventions (Feldman 1994). This allows for teaching of parenting knowledge and skills in either setting, whilst promoting generalisation and maintenance from one setting to another. Parenting requires transfer of learnt skills into new and different situations on a continual basis. This aspect of parenting is particularly difficult for parents with learning disabilities to achieve.

Research has indicated that group interventions are the most cost-effective method of teaching (McGaw 2000). Parenting groups provide useful information to parents with learning disabilities and also an opportunity for the parents to share their stresses and struggles in childrearing. They empower parents by promoting self-esteem, enhancing self-advocacy and increasing parenting skills. The development of social skills and social networks is an important aspect of these groups. As with the home-based teaching programmes, specialised resources and materials are also required for the groups.

SPS provides two parenting groups each year in Cornwall. The location of the groups is dependent on the families' needs. These groups comprise 10 weekly 2-hour sessions. Transportation and crèche facilities are provided. Guest speakers and field trips are an additional feature. The parenting topics are decided upon by the parents themselves and have included:

- emergency responses and safety
- mental health and well-being
- relationships and resources
- stress and relaxation
- behaviour management and play
- assertiveness.

The groups incorporate evidence-based practice, research and evaluation. Pre and post testing determines whether there has been an increase in knowledge and skills. Client evaluations are completed during the final session to provide feedback which will enhance subsequent parenting groups. The high rate of attendance for these groups also indicates their successfulness. The parents' comments on the groups included:

'A break from things/the children'
'Sharing problems'   'Meeting new friends'
'How to help yourself'   'It's given me more self-confidence'
'Listening to others'   'Helped me to speak up at groups'
'Trusting people in the group'   'Helped me to cope'

'Helped me to control the children's behaviour and to control my frustration'

HOW WILL WE KNOW IF OUR PROGRAMME IS SUCCESSFUL?

Evaluating the success of teaching programmes is paramount in addressing the needs of the family and providing continued support. Effective methods of evaluation may include observations, frequency charts, professional feedback, pre and post testing (parent and referrer), parent evaluations, behavioural changes within the family and video feedback. Baseline measures should be taken at the outset of a programme. These can be achieved through assessment, recording of the parent's initial skills, parent documentation, questionnaires and frequency observations. The case study of the Smith family incorporates some of these techniques.

Monitoring and evaluation of teaching programmes further enable identification of areas that need reinforcing and new skills that need to be developed. Careful planning and coordination of services is also critical to ensure that current teaching is reinforced and follow-up support is provided (DoH 2000).

KEY POINTS

- Interventions should be parent centred and focus on the strengths of parents rather than their deficiencies.
- Teaching strategies should be performance based rather than knowledge based and incorporate modelling, practice, feedback and praise.
- Individually tailored, specialised teaching and step-by-step instructions which include visual aids are the most successful training programmes.
- Home-based teaching in conjunction with group interventions leads to generalisation and maintenance of skills and practice.
- Programme monitoring and evaluation must be ongoing throughout the intervention to determine efficacy.
- Coordination of services and collaborative efforts are essential to the success of the intervention. However, it is important to be mindful of not overwhelming families with too many professionals visiting the home and providing services.

REFERENCES

Bakken, J, Miltenberger RG, Schauss S 1993 Teaching parents with mental retardation: knowledge vs. skills. American Journal of Mental Retardation 97: 405–417

Bayley N 1993 Bayley Infant Scales 2. Psychological Corporation, London

Bellman M, Lingham S, Auckett A 1996 Schedule of growing skills, 2nd edn. NFER-Nelson, Windsor

Caldwell BM, Bradley RH 1984 Home observation for measurement of the environment. University of Arkansas, Little Rock, Arkansas

Department of Health, Department of Education and Employment and Home Office 2000 Framework for the Assessment of Children in Need and their Families. DoH, London

Department of Health 2001 Valuing people: a new strategy for learning disability. DoH, London

Espe-Sherwindt M, Kerlin S, Beatty C, Crable S 1990 Parents with special needs/mental retardation: a handbook for early intervention. Project CAPABLE, Handicapped Children's Early Education Program. US Department of Education, Washington DC

Feldman M 1994 Parenting education for parents with intellectual disabilities: a review of outcome studies. Research in Developmental Disabilities 5:299–332

Feldman M, Towns F, Betel J, Case L, Rincover A, Rubino CA 1986 Parent education project 2: increasing stimulating interactions of developmentally handicapped mothers. Journal of Applied Behaviour Analysis 19:23–37

Goodinge S 2000 A jigsaw of services: inspection of services to support disabled adults in their parenting role. Social Services Inspectorate, DoH, London

Horwath J (ed) 2000 The child's world – assessing children in need. DoH, London

Huntley M 1996 Griffiths Mental Development Scales – 1996 Revision. The Test Agency, Henley-on-Thames

Koller H, Richardson SA 1988 Peer relationships of mildly retarded young adults living in the community. Journal of Mental Deficiency 32:321–331

McGaw S 1994 Raising the parental competency of parents with learning disabilities. PhD dissertation

McGaw S 1998 Parents who happen to have a learning disability. In: Emerson E, Caine A, Bromely J, Hatton C (eds) Clinical psychology and people with intellectual disabilities. Wiley, Chichester

McGaw S 2000 What works for parents with learning disabilities? Barnardo's, Ilford, Essex

McGaw S, Sturmey P 1994 Assessing parents with learning disabilities: the parental skills model. Child Abuse Review 3:36–51

McGaw S, Beckley K, Connolly N, Ball D 1998 Parent Assessment Manual. Special Parenting Service, Cornwall and Isles of Scilly Health Authority, Truro

Olsson RH 1994 Ohio Functional Assessment Battery – standardised tests for leisure and living skills. Therapy Skill Builders, Tucson, Arizona

Tymchuk A 1998 The development, implementation and preliminary evaluation of a cross-agency, multi-site, self-healthcare and safety preparation and prevention scheme. School of Medicine, UCLA, California

Tymchuk A, Andron L 1990 Mothers with mental retardation who do or do not abuse or neglect their children. Child Abuse and Neglect 14:313–323

Tymchuk A, Andron L 1992 Project parenting: child interactional training with mothers who are mentally handicapped. Mental Handicap Research 5:4–32

Tymchuk A, Lang C, Dolyniuk C, Ficklin K, Spitz R 1999 The Home Inventory of Dangers and Safety Precautions 2: addressing critical needs for prescriptive assessment devices in child maltreatment and in healthcare. Child Abuse and Neglect 23 (1):1–14

Wechsler D 1988 Wechsler Adult Intelligence Scale – revised. Psychological Corporation, Kent

Young S, Strouthos M 1997 First steps to parenthood. Pavilion, Brighton

RESOURCES

Agencies/National Organisations

Special Parenting Service, 5 Walsingham Place, Truro, Cornwall TR1 2RP.
Tel: 01872 356040
Fax: 01872 356059
Email: Sue.McGaw@cht.swest.nhs.uk
Provides assessments, presentations, training workshops, resources and publications.

Disability, Pregnancy and Parenthood International, National Centre for Disabled Parents, Unit F9, 89–93 Fonthill Road, London N4 3JH.
Helpline: 0800 0184730
Tel: 020 7263 3088
Email: dppi@eotw.co.uk

British Institute for Learning Disabilities (BILD), Wolverhampton Road, Kidderminster, Worcs DY10 3PP.
Tel: 01562 850251
Provides materials, resources, publications, education, training, consultancy, information, research.

Right From the Start, Maternity Alliance, 45 Beech Street, London EC2P 2LX.
Tel: 020 7588 8583 x 133
Email: dquartermaine@maternityalliance.org.uk
Maternity services for parents with LD, advice, support and information.

Disabled Parents Network, Register Coordinator, 36 Meadow View, Pottersbury, Northants NN12 7PH.
National network of disabled people who are parents. Support for people with physical or sensory impairments, long-term illnesses and people with LD.

Values Into Action, Oxford House, Derbyshire Street, London E2 6HG.
Tel: 020 7729 5436
Email: via@btinternet.com
Campaigning organisation working to achieve equal rights for people with LD.

People First, 207–215 Kings Cross Road, London WC1X 9DB.
Tel: 020 7713 6400
Promotes self-advocacy for people with LD.

Parent Support Service, Rounds Green Methodist Church Buildings, Newbury Lane, Oldbury, West Midlands B69 1HE.
Tel: 0121 544 6611
Supports parents with LD in the home.

Homelink, 34 Islington Park Street, London N1 1PX.
Tel: 020 7359 7443
Email: elfrida@elfrida.com.
London-based service supporting parents with LD.

Learning Disabilities Service, Child Protection, Learning Disability Team, Castle Circus Health Centre, Abbey Road, Torquay TQ2 5YH.
Tel: 01803 291231
Early intervention/assessment, training events, support provided by health professionals.

Group Intervention Programmes

Special Parenting Service (see above)

PALS (Parenting, Advocacy, Learning and Support) Project, Ruth Dyson, Project Worker, South Birmingham FSU, 45 Barratts Road, Birmingham B38 9HU.
Tel: 0121 4594232

Email: sbfu@virgin.net
Home-based support, teaching, and groupwork.

Life Programme (University of Illinois, 1987). Developmental Services Center, 1304 W. Bradley Avenue, Champaign, Illinois 61821.

Books and other resources

Feldman M, Case L 1992 Step-by-step: a manual for parents and childcare providers. Available from Dr Maurice Feldman, Department of Psychology, Queen's University, Kingston, Ontario, Canada K71 3N6.
Tel: (613) 545-2491.
Email: feldman@psyc.queensu.ca

Parenting booklets and parenting skill cards (McGaw et al 1995–99).
Available from BILD (see above).

Red Cross 1988 Parenting: birth to six for parents with special learning needs. Red Cross, USA.

Needs jigsaw. Silverdale 1999. Available from 17 Durkar Fields, Wakefield WF4 3BY.

Matthews DR 1996 The OK Health Check. Assessing and planning the health care need of people with LD. Available from Fairfield Publications, PO Box 310, Preston Central PR1 9GH.

Beu D 1999 Thumbs up! An assertiveness training pack. Available from Pavilion Publishing, 8 St George's Place, Brighton, East Sussex BN1 4GB.

McIntosh P, O'Neil J 1999 Food, fitness, and fun. Training pack in weight management for people with LD. Available from Pavilion Publishing, 8 St George's Place, Brighton, East Sussex BN1 4GB.

10 Supporting parents of children who are disabled

Mary Nolan

This chapter is based on an interview with Sue, the mother of Sarah (9 years old) who has Down's syndrome, and Lindsey, the mother of Daniel (11 years old) who has cerebral palsy. I am immensely indebted to these two women who shared with me their experiences and insights. Both felt strongly that they were the people who knew their children best and who were in the best position to make decisions about their care and education. What they needed from health professionals was not advice on how to bring their children up but empowerment to help them work 'the system' and use information from a variety of sources to make the best possible decisions for their children. Health professionals can either undermine parents' confidence in parenting their children with disabilities or empower parents to become equal partners with them. When accepted as equal partners, parents are in a strong position to help their children take their place in society.

Mary (Interviewer): *Please tell me a little about your children and how you felt when you found out that they had a disability.*

Lindsey: I can remember the Friday morning when the consultant told me that Daniel had cerebral palsy. For months, I had thought he was gradually recovering from the meningitis he contracted when he was 6 months old. The diagnosis came out of the blue. Although I was profoundly shocked, I can remember making an immediate decision right then, in the room with the consultant, that I wanted to help my child. I didn't want my child looked after by other people because I didn't know what to do for him myself. I wanted the professionals to help me to learn how to help him.

Sue: Yes – when I was told that Sarah had Down's syndrome, I was shocked. I just felt a desperate need to go home, away from the hospital and away from all the people talking at me and trying to do things for me. I wanted to sort out for myself how I was going to manage this situation. My world had just fallen apart and my emotions were out of control. I needed time to adjust to the fact that, suddenly, the whole world was seeing my child as a disabled child and me as the parent of a disabled child. That really undermines your confidence – the assumption that all normality has now gone from your life and that you and your child are totally different from other parents and children. I needed the reassurance that I was a normal parent and I wanted information about the things that my child could and would be able to do. I knew perfectly well that my child wouldn't reach developmental milestones at the same time as other children but I did want to have a rough idea of when she might reach them. And she has reached them – it's just taken a little longer than normal.

Lindsey: That's exactly how I felt. The disability gets in the way of the child. Daniel isn't a 'cerebral palsy child'; he's a child with cerebral palsy. I want the child to be acknowledged before the disability and then everyone can focus on him as an individual rather than as a case history. It's awful when people talk about 'these children'. Daniel isn't one of 'these children'. He's unique.

Sue: That's right. When Sarah was diagnosed and we started having input from lots of different professionals, I was scared to death that all they would do was *train* her to do things, rather than help her to make decisions and choose what she wanted to do.

Mary (Interviewer): What do parents need from health professionals when they find out that their child has a disability?

Lindsey: What you need is reassurance that the stuff you already know about babies and children still applies. When you're told that your child has cerebral palsy or Down's syndrome, everything you know about children goes out of the window. You don't know whether you can do the ordinary things with your child that other parents do. You need permission to behave normally and play with your child and talk to him and do all the things that you'd have done if he'd not had a disability.

Sue: Because the child *is* normal in so many respects. Just as you're normal parents making decisions for your child like any other parents. It's just that your decisions have an extra dimension. You have the same aspirations for your disabled child as you do for their siblings or as any other parents would have for their children. But you have to accept that it will take longer to realise them and you may have to go by a different route.

Lindsey: You need health professionals to treat you in such a way that you feel like an equal partner. When health professionals treat you like a normal parent, you are empowered to feel and behave and think like a normal parent. It can be exhausting with so many appointments to see so many health professionals. And everyone seems to focus on what your child can't do, rather than on what he can do. I needed to hear my child praised occasionally. I wanted to be a normal parent. I had the same needs as any other parent.

Sue: It's really easy to lose sight of the fact that you're a normal parent. When you have a child with a disability, you're overwhelmed with health professionals wanting to input into the child's 'management'. Paediatricians, physiotherapists, speech therapists, child psychologists, GPs, midwives, health visitors – they all want to have their say, which is valuable if they can see themselves *as only part of the picture*. There are always other professionals with different ideas and suggestions. The speech therapist might suggest an activity to be practised every day. The occupational therapist suggests a 15-minute set of exercises, three times a day. The visiting teacher suggests a sorting activity twice a day. This is overwhelming – it needs coordinating so that you have space to feel like a normal parent.

Lindsey: What you want as parents is to be consulted, to work through various options, discuss different ways of achieving certain goals and then decide what will best suit your child and your family circumstances. It isn't helpful just to be *told* what to do, because if you can't manage, you feel you have failed your child and the professional concerned. There are enough negative emotions without adding to them.

Mary (Interviewer): *How important is continuity of carer?*

Sue: You need to see the same person from each health profession, so that you can establish a relationship and you don't have to explain your child's condition over and over. Explaining things again and again in the early days is very upsetting and makes you feel even more vulnerable. I wanted to see the same midwife, the same health visitor, the same paediatrician. I used to ring the clinic in advance and if my health visitor wasn't going to be on that afternoon, I'd cancel my appointment and say I'd wait until she was next available to see me.

Mary (Interviewer): *What about support groups?*

Sue: Health professionals can encourage you to meet other parents with children who have Down's syndrome. And you do need some encouragement to begin with. In the early days, I felt sick at the thought of being in a room with lots of children who had Down's syndrome, seeing them at 2 years old and 3 years old and having a vision of what my baby would be like when she was that old. And the first time I went to a group, I couldn't even look at the children. When I got home, my husband wanted to know what the children were like who were older than Sarah. But I couldn't tell him because I hadn't looked at them!

Lindsey: But you just have to keep on going. And parents with children like yours are the ones who can tell you what you really need to know – such as how to get the allowances you're entitled to and how to arrange Portage and about seeing the social worker. It's invaluable.

Mary (Interviewer): *How were you helped to educate your children when they were small?*

Sue: We had portage through an organisation called KIDS*. A Portage advisor came to see me and Sarah every week, 52 weeks a year, for one to one and a half hours. She really got to know us and I felt I could tell her the truth about how things were and expose my feelings to her because I had built up such a good relationship with her. She really understood how much effort Sarah and I had to put in to achieve certain things. And she celebrated Sarah's achievements and helped me celebrate them, however small they were. I could share the high points with her. I couldn't share them as fully with other people because they didn't understand what it meant to us.

Lindsey: A really good visiting advisor empowers you to coordinate your life. For example, you are given a weekly 9 am appointment at the hospital for a therapy session. Initially, your life is totally disrupted in order to keep that appointment. Siblings have to have alternative arrangements made for getting them to school. Baby has to have his morning routine completely altered and he's upset as a result. The traffic is horrendous. You're stressed, but you feel that 'I can't change it – it's a HOSPITAL APPOINTMENT!' The advisor then suggests to you that it's OK to make a phone call to the hospital to discuss another time for the appointment. A 10.30 appointment is arranged and the result is that you're happier, the children are happier, the baby's contented and you have a more successful therapy session. Sometimes, it's possible to arrange for the speech therapist or health visitor to visit while the Portage

---

* Contact details for KIDS can be found at the end of Chapter 4.

worker is at your house. So everyone starts to get a truer picture of how the child is progressing.

Mary (Interviewer): *What are the key points for health professionals helping parents with children who are disabled to be good-enough parents?*

Sue: You have to be strong to be the parent of a child who has a disability and health professionals can help you to be strong. They can let you be in control instead of having to be in control themselves. They can empower you to become a partner in decision making so that you can make informed decisions. It's not about who's in control – it's about ensuring the best choices are made for your child.

Lindsey: It really makes me angry when I hear that information has been kept back from parents or when health professionals don't communicate with each other about your child. You need to be kept fully in the picture so that you can make the best decisions for your child. You know him better than anyone. When you are kept informed and have things explained to you, then you grow as a parent and you can give your child the best possible parenting.

Sue: The parent is like a managing director. The MD needs the correct information, on time, from each department, if she is going to make the right commercial decisions for the company. The parent also needs all the facts, communicated in a professional manner, in the timespan agreed. Then she can make the best decisions for her child. It's important not to burden parents with thinking too far in advance. Help parents to take one day at a time and celebrate the child's achievements at that point. Don't present too many issues in one go. Help parents think through one issue before going onto the next.

Lindsey: It's true, though, that parents *are* very concerned with the future and do need some questions answering, but it's important that health professionals should say they don't know if they don't. Help parents link what you're doing with what other health professionals are doing. This needs some joined-up thinking because health professionals often don't seem to communicate with each other at all. The speech therapist needs to know what the health visitor is doing and so on, so that there's a coordinated approach to the child and parents can understand what's happening and what part they play.

Sue: Show that you trust the parents. Ask them what the child can do and what she can't do. And then start from that point. Remember that the parent is the first and most important educator of their child.

Lindsey: Try and involve other family members in what you're doing to make the point that this child is part of a whole family. That helps the child feel good and it helps the parents feel that their family is OK. It's important to remember that the child with the disability is not the sole focus of the family – there are other family members with their own needs.

Mary (Interviewer): *Sometimes health professionals say that parents of children who are disabled are pushy and aggressive. Is that true, do you think?*

Sue: Maybe it is. But the question you have to ask is *why* the parents feel they need to be so assertive. Perhaps it's because they've had such bad experiences in the past, of being kept in the dark or talked down to or not trusted, that they have learned to be distrustful. Let me give you an example. An ENT consultant is talking to the mother of a 3-year-old child with Down's syndrome. The child's hearing is poor and the mother is trying to establish what options there are for treatment. The consultant speaks in this manner:

> Well, you see, these children often have problems... These children tend to have very small ear canals...These children tend not to tolerate hearing aids.

Eventually, the mother asks, 'Do you mean all 3 year olds or all children with poor hearing or all children with Down's syndrome? If my child did not have Down's syndrome, what treatment would you suggest to improve her hearing?' As you can imagine, repeated encounters of this nature result in the family requesting a different consultant!

Lindsey: Ultimately, it is a question of acknowledging and respecting the fact that the parent is the most knowledgeable person about that child. Education is to do with making parents feel good about themselves and their children. Everyone has a valuable input, but they need to work in partnership with the parents to fulfil the child's potential.

Sue: Above all, I really want health professionals to be open and honest with me. I want them to send signals to me that they consider me to be someone who is capable of looking after my child and capable of making good decisions for her. Parents need to be empowered and health professionals have enormous influence on whether you feel empowered or totally helpless.

Lindsey: I do need support while I am bringing up my child and, of course, I am grateful for the specialist input that Daniel has. But, at the end of the day, I am also an expert about my child and I'm the one who's going to coordinate his care and make most of the decisions about him.

KEY POINTS

- Acknowledge the child before the disability. Acknowledge the parents as parents first and parents of a child with extra needs second.
- Empower parents who have a child with a disability to make the best use of the health and social services available to them.
- Help them to assert themselves and to explain the need, as far as is reasonable, for continuity of carer.
- Explore with the parents what information they need and help them obtain it.
- Empower parents to make their own decisions for their child.
- Celebrate what the child can do, rather than considering only what s/he can't.

AFTERWORD: RESOURCES

The two mothers whom I interviewed both felt that health visitors are vital in helping families whose baby has been born with a disability to find information. Midwives visit for 10 days and they are the ones who see the 'grief period'.

After that, one of the most frequent ports of call is the baby clinic for regular weighing sessions. Health visitors could contact a relevant charity for information, e.g. Scope, Down's Syndrome Association, Mencap, etc., and have everything ready to give to the parents.

Relevant and up-to-date information is often very hard for parents to find in the early stages of diagnosis. Even if they are given a phone number or address, it can be very hard to pursue. It is often more helpful to be given the information which someone else has obtained. Feelings of paralysis and an inability to do even simple things such as make phone calls is common when people are in shock. Health visitors are in a key position to advise families of local services available within the statutory sectors of health, education and social services and, equally importantly, within the voluntary sector.

11 Parenting education for women in prison

Denise Marshall

INTRODUCTION

A woman's experience of pregnancy, labour and parenting can be significantly different because she is in prison. This chapter concentrates on what is particular to the experience of parenting in prison. It is based on my experience of teaching antenatal classes in Holloway Prison and on the baby massage and postnatal support sessions that I offer to mothers on the Mother and Baby Unit there.

The number of women in prison has been rising rapidly. In 1992–93 the average number of women in prison during any month was 1374 (Prison Reform Trust website, January 2001). By the end of January 1999, this had increased to 3187. The majority of these were mothers (61%) each having, on average, two children under the age of 18 (Howard League for Penal Reform 1999).

Four prisons in England and Wales provide Mother and Baby Units with a total of 64 places for babies. Places at Holloway Mother and Baby Unit are for babies up to nine months old. Mothers can then apply to be transferred to Styal or Askham Grange prisons where babies can remain with them until 18 months old. There are currently no places for older infants in the prison service. The Howard League estimated in February 1999 that as many as 600 children under two years old were being affected by the imprisonment of their mothers.

Mothers arrive on Mother and Baby Units in prison at different stages of motherhood. Most of the mothers on the Holloway Mother and Baby Unit have come to prison while pregnant and have given birth at a local hospital, accompanied by prison officers. Some women, however, begin their imprisonment with their baby, having already begun their parenting outside prison, while others have transferred from another prison where mother and baby facilities do not exist. In either of these situations, there is often a temporary separation of mother and baby from a few hours to a couple of weeks.

Some mothers and babies spend only a few weeks on a Mother and Baby Unit because the mother has a short sentence or is in prison on remand and is then found not guilty when her case comes to court. Most spend a longer period and will perhaps do all their early parenting in prison. Some will also face transfer to a new prison before the baby reaches nine months old and some will be separated from their baby at 18 months old when the baby is either 'handed out' to family or is placed in the care of Social Services.

Women who go to prison are likely to have a greater need for care and support than other women. They are more likely to have spent time in care during childhood (25% of women in Holloway in 1993–94) or to have been victims of abuse (again, 25% in 1993–94) than women in the community. It has been estimated that 56% of women in prison have mental health problems (Prison Reform Trust 2001). They are more likely to have a history of drug or alcohol abuse or to have tried to harm themselves in the past than women in the non-prison population.

MOTHERS' ANTENATAL EXPERIENCE

Women who are pregnant and in prison are probably experiencing quite a different preparation for parenthood from mothers in the community.

Women describe missing a sense of 'specialness' that they had felt being pregnant outside prison. They talk about the 'loss' that they feel in not being looked after by their mother or their partner because they are not at home. Women have talked to me in antenatal classes about particular dishes cooked for them in a previous pregnancy, cravings for foods not available in prison and massages that they would be having if they were at home. Prison meal times and routines do not make allowances for morning sickness and heartburn; it is difficult to eat little and often in prison. Being in prison makes it extremely difficult for a woman to respond to the changes taking place in her body during pregnancy: to eat or not to eat, to sleep, to lie down, put her feet up when she feels necessary. Some women also find it difficult coping with the emotional ups and downs of pregnancy in prison where 'snapping' at an officer or another prisoner could lead to a loss of privileges such as phone calls home. More positively, imprisonment during pregnancy might provide some women with the opportunity to come off drugs or to break with a stressful and damaging lifestyle. It may be a respite from 'normal' life and the chance to receive antenatal care that they might not otherwise have had. They may feel more 'cared for' in prison because of this and enjoy the support of other prisoners. Nevertheless, they will still be experiencing frustrations and anxieties that arise from the loss of liberty during pregnancy.

Pregnant women in prison, not surprisingly, report feeling high levels of anxiety and depression. Some women are on remand awaiting trial (approximately three-quarters of prisoners in Holloway) while others may have already been convicted but are awaiting sentencing and do not know whether they will be released before or after their baby is born. Other women, who may know that they will be in prison when their baby is born, are waiting to hear whether they will have a place on the Mother and Baby Unit.

An antenatal clinic for pregnant women in Holloway is run three mornings a week by three midwives from the Whittington Hospital on the unit (C4) where most pregnant women are housed. The women say that as the midwives are not part of the prison, they treat them as pregnant women rather than as prisoners, which they greatly appreciate. These midwives provide continuity of care in pregnancy and although women do not necessarily see one of them during labour, they do always receive a visit postnatally. A weekly antenatal class is also held on C4 (currently run by myself) which covers preparation for labour and early parenthood. The class provides an opportunity for women to talk about their feelings and anxieties about being pregnant in prison, about the labour and what will happen once they have had the baby. Women have said that the chance to practise 'breathing' and massage and watch birth videos in the classes has helped them to feel more like a pregnant woman on the 'outside' and to focus on their baby. Mothers who have already had their baby and are on the Mother and Baby Unit are encouraged to visit the antenatal class to talk about their labour, their baby and life on the Mother and Baby Unit.

This link between the antenatal classes on C4 and the Mother and Baby Unit works well in a number of ways. Fears about going into labour in prison, being accompanied to hospital by officers and raising a baby on the Mother and Baby Unit can to some extent be allayed by the visiting mothers. Pregnant women, particularly those having their first baby, can learn from seeing babies of different ages being fed, changed, played with, etc. They meet existing mothers, to whom they may be able to turn later for support on the Mother and Baby Unit, once they have had their babies. Returning to the antenatal classes to 'tell their story' is also empowering for the women who have recently become mothers. They are able to give information to the class about the Mother and Baby Unit and what it is like to look after a baby there. They are seen as the 'experts' on looking after a baby on the Unit.

Information about breastfeeding is given by a supporter from the Breastfeeding Network who holds an antenatal class every five or six weeks. It is particularly important to adapt this to the needs of the pregnant women in prison. If they will be in prison with their babies, most mothers want to be reassured that breastfeeding will not prevent them from 'handing their baby out' for short visits to the father and/or other family members. The breastfeeding supporter explains how to express milk and shows mothers the electric pump available for use on the Mother and Baby Unit; she also talks about 'mixed feeding'. Many mothers will be returning to 'work' in the prison by the time their baby is six weeks old, if not earlier, because of economic necessity. Some mothers rely on their prison wages to buy nappies and essentials for the baby; this is the case with foreign nationals and mothers who are not being economically supported by their family. Child benefit does not arrive for several weeks and mothers in prison are not entitled to other benefits, so these women need information on how breastfeeding can be combined with 2–3 hour work sessions in prison.

Women who have not breastfed other children, or who had not intended to breastfeed this baby, have decided to breastfeed because of the information they have gained in antenatal classes. Women feel encouraged to 'give breastfeeding a try' because of meeting the supporter antenatally and knowing that she can visit them once they are feeding their baby. The supporter usually visits the Mother and Baby Unit once a week and can be contacted by phone. Breastfeeding mothers from the Mother and Baby Unit visit the antenatal classes and provide a strong peer group image for mothers considering breastfeeding.

There is often a majority of mothers on the unit breastfeeding for the first six weeks, but there are a number of women whose ability to breastfeed does seem to be affected by the stress of being in prison. Encouragement and support for breastfeeding in this environment must be balanced with tact and sensitivity towards women's vulnerability and personal choices. It has to be remembered that a higher proportion of women in prison than in the community are HIV positive or taking medication which is contraindicated while breastfeeding. These women often need support in coming to terms with the fact that they will not breastfeed.

MOTHERS' EXPERIENCE OF LABOUR

There is much anxiety around going into labour in prison. Labouring women are taken by ambulance (or occasionally minicab) to a local designated hospital. Security considerations mean that pregnant prisoners do not previously visit the labour ward, as pregnant women in the community are encouraged to do. Women are most likely to go into labour in the evening or night-time when they are locked in their cell. Different procedures apply at different prisons, but the officer on duty usually waits to have labour confirmed by a member of the prison's medical staff before calling an ambulance. Because the pregnant woman is a prisoner, the decision about when to go to hospital is not in her hands. Although it is rarely a problem, most women worry about how long they will have to wait for an officer to respond to their buzzer when they are in labour and how quickly they will then get to hospital.

The labouring woman is almost always accompanied to hospital by two uniformed officers who wait outside the delivery room, unless asked to be present by the woman. However, if the woman is not in established labour but needs to be in hospital, the officers are then, for security reasons, stationed by the hospital bed on 'bedwatch'. Some women in this situation who might be in early labour, having their labour induced or awaiting a caesarean section will receive support from their accompanying officer, particularly if they have had the chance to establish a relationship with her beforehand.

Other women describe feeling embarrassed in front of the other pregnant women on the ward and unable to relax in the presence of the officers, one of whom could be male.

A labouring woman prisoner may be some distance, even hundreds of miles from the partner, family member or friend whom she would like to support her in labour. There are only five women's prisons in England and Wales which receive prisoners on remand and Holloway takes prisoners from 240 courts in 14 counties (Wurr 1998).

Women can have the birth partner/s of their choice at the hospital but rely on the prison to contact them when they go into labour. This can be a considerable cause of concern antentally as women worry whether their birth partner will be contacted and then able to get to the hospital in time.

One important source of support for women in prison is the Association for Women Facing Childbirth in Detention (a registered charity). Members of the Association are antenatal teachers, midwives and others committed to supporting women in labour. They are available as birth companions for women from Holloway going into hospital to give birth. There are a number of reasons why women prisoners may need a birth companion. They may be foreign nationals without friends or family in this country; their partner may also be in prison; family and friends may live too far away to get to the hospital in time or they may be estranged from their families. Members of the Association visit antenatally and talk through a birth plan with women who are interested in having a birth companion. The birth companion is there to offer support in whatever way the labouring woman chooses and may only be needed until the woman's family arrives. Many women have said that having this support in labour and after the birth made them feel 'special' and 'cared for' and helped them to cope with their situation as a prisoner in labour. Birth companions also visit mothers on the Mother and Baby Unit postnatally and can form part of the support network that mothers in prison need to establish.

It is understandable that a pregnant woman prisoner may well be very anxious during her pregnancy and find it difficult to relax. In labour she may find it hard to focus on her contractions, listen to her body and go with the flow, particularly if she has had a long period of being 'guarded' in early labour. Some women have positive experiences of labour and birth and feel supported by their birth partner/s, midwives and sometimes by their accompanying officers. However, there are undoubtedly many women who experience feelings of disempowerment, humiliation and anxiety during labour as a result of being a prisoner. They may be left with feelings of 'loss' and disappointment about their pregnancy and birth experience.

EARLY PARENTING IN PRISON

Mothers with new babies in prison have many of the same needs as any new mother in the community. Their questions and concerns are very similar, as is their need to be supported and to gain confidence in the care of their new baby.

Most mothers on the Holloway Mother and Baby Unit have had antenatal and birth experiences which have been significantly affected by being a prisoner. A mother in this situation may have a great need to talk about her experience of pregnancy and birth and to 'debrief' before she can begin to focus on her baby. The transition from hospital and back to prison with a new baby can be a difficult one and may coincide with the time when the new mother is already feeling vulnerable and 'weepy' as her milk comes in. Support and practical help in these first few days are vital in enabling the mother to gain confidence in her ability to feed and look after her baby. A mother in prison has been removed from her familiar surroundings and from her support structure of family and friends. In prison, she needs to build an alternative support network for herself based on other mothers and women in the prison, health professionals, those working with her in various roles and officers. It is important that support is available from several sources so that mothers can choose to confide in the people they feel most comfortable with.

There is a whole range of people who might form part of this support network in addition to the midwives, antenatal teacher, breastfeeding supporter and birth companions already mentioned. A health visitor visits the Unit weekly, providing the sort of support and information that mothers would usually get at the community baby clinic. A core of officers works regularly on the Unit and gets to know the mothers and babies. A group of volunteers from a local church comes in twice a week and can take babies out in their buggies for a walk, if their mothers wish, to accustom them to 'outside' noises and to get baby shopping for the mothers. Two nursery nurses run a crèche for the babies on the Unit, mainly for when mothers are working or taking education courses. They provide a role model of how to play with infants and their example of 'how to be' with a baby can be influential. Some women are also visited by the prison chaplains or request a visit from a 'befriender', a prisoner who has volunteered to offer support to other women in Holloway.

SUPPORT FROM OTHER MOTHERS

Mothers on the Unit can also provide an enormous amount of support for each other. Mothers with babies who are crying a lot in the first three months are often helped by other mothers who look after the crying baby to give the mother a break. This can be particularly necessary during the 12–15 hours, evening-to-morning stretch when mothers have to stay in their rooms. Although not 'locked in' (because the baby is not a prisoner), mothers and babies must stay behind their doors for the same periods as other prisoners at Holloway. However, officers can be asked to take a crying baby down the corridor to another mother and sometimes officers will look after the baby to give the mother a break. This time 'behind the doors' can be particularly difficult for a new mother with a crying baby and also for mothers with older babies who are starting to be mobile and feel frustrated by the lack of space and variety in the very small rooms.

Experienced mothers tend to show new mothers how to bath their baby and carry out other babycare tasks and the atmosphere can be very supportive. However, this is not every mother's experience of the Unit. Some women feel isolated or may be bullied, depending on the atmosphere and mix of women at any particular time.

OPPORTUNITIES FOR LEARNING PARENTING SKILLS

Women on the Mother and Baby Unit have generally had the opportunity to cover aspects of parenting at the C4 antenatal and breast feeding classes. They may also have had some antenatal contact with mothers and babies from the Unit and talked about parenting issues. Once women have had their babies, a great deal of informal parentcraft learning occurs during the contact that mothers have with all the people mentioned previously.

It is at first surprising that mothers on the Holloway Mother and Baby Unit, who are receptive to talking about their baby on a one-to-one basis, are often reluctant to come to either an informal mother and baby group or a more formal parentcraft class. However, an important difference between mothers in prison and those in the community is that mothers on the Unit are not motivated to come to a group or class by the need to meet other women and share experiences of parenting. They are surrounded by mothers and are unlikely to need to talk with them about baby issues any more than they are doing already. Some mothers may be feeling the need for greater privacy with their baby or may actively wish to avoid contact with particular mothers because of the inevitable personality clashes and differences that result from women living so closely together. It is clear that most mothers are already receiving some form of peer group support and that isolation is not a primary issue.

Another barrier to bringing mothers together to discuss parentcraft is the general reluctance amongst women in Holloway to be open about feelings and experiences unless they are with trusted people. This is more marked on the Mother and Baby Unit than amongst the pregnant women on C4, possibly because mothers feel that they have more to lose. Women on the Unit express worries about whether officers and other mothers perceive them to be coping, particularly if they have a baby who cries more than average or if they are feeling depressed and finding looking after their baby difficult. Women who have been interviewed to determine whether they are 'suitable' for the Unit and who know that their place is conditional on 'good' behaviour worry about gossip and malicious reports and there is a feeling of being observed when they are with their baby. An incident such as a baby rolling off the bed, which would be viewed as 'normal', though upsetting, for a mother in the community and might be talked about by her in a postnatal group, would be seen differently by women in prison. A mother on the Mother and Baby Unit might well feel too apprehensive to share her distress about this with anyone else.

Various kinds of parentcraft classes have been run in the Unit in recent years. The problem of attendance has usually been dealt with by making a certain number of classes compulsory, as part of the contract when mothers accept their place on the Mother and Baby Unit. Another method that has helped to ensure attendance is providing baby 'freebies' for mothers attending classes, such as bibs and beakers. The classes have tended to be more information than discussion based because of the reasons mentioned earlier. They have generally been run by the nursery nurses who work on the Unit Monday to Friday, together with the health visitor and antenatal teacher from C4.

Having a range of people running the sessions with different teaching styles has worked well. As the C4 antenatal teacher, I have offered baby massage sessions, alternating with the more information-based sessions, and this has been successful. However, I do not feel completely comfortable with the compulsory nature of the classes. Others working on the parentcraft course feel the compulsory element is necessary because of the apathy created in mothers by being in prison and their disinclination to come together in a group. Some mothers feel it should be their choice whether or not to attend parentcraft classes.

Usually, more than half the mothers on the Unit have at least one older child. Although the experience of these mothers can be very useful in a parentcraft class, difficulties can arise when mothers recommend methods which conflict with current advice; for example, regarding when to introduce solids and different sleeping positions. This situation needs to be handled sensitively in a way that does not negate the mother's experiences and alienate her from the classes. A separate class for first-time mothers could work well. A current plan is to introduce parentcraft classes which include practical sessions such as mobile making, to appeal to both first-time and experienced mothers. Mothers in prison worry that their babies are being deprived of the normal experiences of babyhood and material things. Therefore, most mothers are highly motivated to make things for their babies and to resume work shortly after the birth so that they can provide toys and clothes. Being able to make things so that her cell is attractive and stimulating for her baby would encourage a mother to attend parentcraft classes. Another incentive being considered is to award a certificate for attendance.

For the past three years, I have been teaching baby massage on the Mother and Baby Unit and have experimented with a variety of formats to try to maximise the numbers of mothers taking part. I began with the approach that I had used successfully in the community, namely mothers massaging their babies while I demonstrated on a doll. After the massage, chat about sleep, feeding and other babycare issues followed naturally in the community classes. This model has worked from time to time in Holloway when I have had a small group of mothers who previously attended my antenatal classes and have already formed themselves into a support group. However, a new mother joining the group or a mother starting prison work might change the dynamics so that the others would no longer attend. Most mothers seem to prefer an individual, one-to-one massage session in their rooms which gives rise to a freer discussion of parenting or other issues which the mother needs to talk about. I now offer baby massage over the lunchtime so that it is available for mothers who are otherwise working. For some mothers who are not receiving any assistance from their family or any other source, working takes priority over all other activities.

Learning to massage her baby can help a mother to feel that she is giving him something special and to feel less anxious about her baby 'missing out' because she is in prison. It can also help a mother to bond with and feel more confident in handling her baby in an environment which can instill passivity, with mothers living according to a routine that is not their own. A mother can massage her baby irrespective of her financial situation (I provide massage oil) and it is a resource for the mother to draw on during the evenings when mother and baby are alone together in their room.

The concerns raised by mothers when seen on a one-to-one basis show that they are often preoccupied with matters arising out of their situation as a parent in prison rather than the more usual postnatal worries. Mothers often want to talk about their other children: how these children are coping with the separation, how they are doing at school and how they may feel about the new baby. Mothers are also worried about whether the father and/or other children will be able to bond with the baby at a later stage and how their own relationship with the baby's father will be affected by the separation and the new baby.

Mothers may be having difficulties with family looking after older children. One new mother, with a six-year-old girl being looked after by her family, was very unhappy because they would not bring her for visits to the prison. She had not seen her daughter for several months. Another mother was very worried about her teenage son who had dropped out of college and been in trouble with the police while she was in prison; she felt that this would not have happened had she been at home. Mothers who are coming up to their trial or sentencing may want to talk about this. The length of their sentence may determine whether they have to be separated from their baby and whether their baby will be placed with Social Services if they do not have someone on the outside to care for him. Mothers who are going home soon may be anxious about where they will be living or about facing problems that they left behind when they came into prison.

The usual concerns about a baby's health appear to be magnified in prison because of the mother's loss of liberty and restricted access to medical attention. A mother cannot just take her baby to the clinic, to her GP or to a hospital casualty department in the middle of the night if she is worried, but must put in a request to see a doctor. Medical care is provided by doctors and nurses based in Holloway and employed by the Prison Service. Many mothers feel that they are treated differently from how they would be in the community and that their fears are not taken seriously. The worry about not getting proper medical care for the baby if needed, combined with the fact that mothers spend long periods alone with their babies, does seem to give rise to increased anxieties about the baby's health. One mother, who already had several children, said that she had been much more anxious about this baby than the previous ones. She felt that she had not been able to find her own rhythm of doing things because of the prison routines and worried about things that she had not noticed with her other children because of the long evenings she spent alone with her baby. Only with this baby had she had problems with breastfeeding.

KEY POINTS

- Mothers may experience a prison Mother and Baby Unit very differently depending on their character, circumstances, recent experiences, feelings and also the particular mix of women on the Unit at the time.
- Some mothers in prison feel more able to relax with their baby and breastfeed successfully because of having support and not having to look after other children and manage the household.
- Some women enjoy the friendship of other mothers, which they might not have had at home.
- Some feel isolated and that they share nothing in common with the other mothers on the Unit.
- Some mothers say that they find it hard to cope and to be a mother because of prison restrictions and routines.
- Some experience a deep sense of injustice at being in prison with a baby and feel that the baby and their other children are being punished as well as themselves.
- Some worry that the baby may suffer developmentally because of the prison environment.
- Supporting and educating women in prison requires a good understanding of the prison environment and of the particular pressures affecting women who are mothering in prison.

REFERENCES

Howard League for Penal Reform 1999 Call to end the imprisonment of babies. 10th February. http://www.penlex.org.uk/pages/hlmbu99.html

Prison Reform Trust 2001 Women in prison: recent trends and developments. http://www.penlex.org.uk/pages/prthigh.html

Wurr M (Chair of Board of Visitors) 1998 Women are different. HMP Holloway, National Advisory Council Newsheet, August, p 2. http://www.penlex.org.uk/pages/nac0304.html

12 Support and information needs of parents with children conceived through assisted conception

Olivia Montuschi

Difficulties with conceiving a child are increasing. As women choose or are forced by economic circumstances to postpone childbearing and sperm counts around the developed world plummet, as many as one in seven couples are likely to find themselves seeking help in starting or adding to their family.

Whether the fertility issue lies with the male or the female partner or is unexplained, the effect of *prolonged* infertility on a relationship is life changing, with a proportion of couples brought closer together by the experience and a number being driven apart.

It is now recognised that the experience of infertility, particularly if it has involved many invasive treatments and/or long periods of doubt and uncertainty about ever achieving a pregnancy, is not necessarily completely resolved by the birth of a healthy child. Because lengthy infertility can colour pregnancy, birth and subsequent parenting, this chapter starts with the range of feelings experienced by men and women as they confront fundamental issues of sex, money and loss of control in a wholly unanticipated way. It continues through the investigation and treatment phase to pregnancy, birth, the transition to parenthood and longer term issues, examining at each stage the feelings and needs of the people involved and how the professionals they encounter can best help to support and inform them on their journey.

In order to be able to offer appropriate information and support, it is helpful for professionals to understand something of the experience of couples who are expecting a baby or parenting children following significant difficulties with conception. Even more important is the willingness and capacity of professionals to reflect upon their own feelings, beliefs and experiences of assisted conception. Negative or mixed feelings are not 'wrong' but need to be acknowledged and high-quality supervision sought if the professional feels that her or his ability to offer genuine support may be at risk of being compromised.

'I DON'T SEEM TO BE GETTING PREGNANT, DOCTOR'

When a couple have been trying for some time without success to conceive a child, the usual first port of call when they decide to seek help is their GP. It is often the female partner who attends by herself first, possibly assuming or even hoping that the problem, if there is one, is hers. In fact, this first consultation may have been delayed because of unwillingness by one or both partners to acknowledge that anything might be wrong, particularly if guilt about past behaviour, infections or an abortion is part of the background. They may also be reluctant to acknowledge that conception at a time of their choosing seems to have moved beyond their control and that carefully planned life stages are not working out as they hoped. These, or other anxieties, are likely to be lingering in the background and a response which acknowledges in a general way the distress that inability to conceive can cause can go a long way to normalising feelings and freeing a couple to take part in any plan to address the situation. Willingness on the part of a GP to take appropriate action in consultation with the couple is also a vital component of support.

WHEN TEST RESULTS COME THROUGH

Initial tests on the male partner's semen and to determine a woman's hormone levels are often done through the GP service. Indications that one or other partner is unlikely to be able to fulfil their role in making a baby without significant medical intervention may become clarified at this stage. Referral to a specialist fertility unit is now advisable. In the meantime, GPs, practice nurses or counsellors attached to a GP practice have a significant part to play in listening to the feelings of the couple and helping them begin to address the range of emotions and issues they are likely to have to face, both individually and together. It can be very helpful for couples to know that men and women often respond very differently to news of infertility. Patricia Irwin Johnston, in her book *Taking Charge of Infertility* (1994), says, 'Men tend to be inclined to look for logical answers, women tend to feel things from the heart. Men tend to be less inclined to share their innermost fears and women are more inclined to spill them all for many to see and hear'. Women can feel abandoned by a partner who needs to grieve quietly or perhaps search the Internet for answers and men can feel overwhelmed by their partner's need to talk. Reflecting on this can help couples begin to understand and respect the way the other partner is handling the situation.

THE ISSUE OF LOSS

Even if the couple are eventually able to become parents, using their own or donated gametes (eggs, embryos or sperm), through surrogacy or by adoption, the issue of loss often remains: the loss of dreams, the loss of privacy, the loss of control over many aspects of life during treatment, loss of spontaneity in lovemaking, loss of time whilst concentrating on infertility, loss of the possibility of having the child of a loved partner, loss of genetic continuity. Although many of these losses can be accommodated and integrated into life over time, they are rarely completely forgotten. One mother of a child conceived by donor insemination commented:

> It was really only when our son was seven or eight and I was having difficulty getting on with him that I realised how much I had wanted a child who

looked like my husband and had his qualities. Once I had realised this and grieved again for the child we could not have together, I was able to recognise and appreciate the many wonderful qualities our son has and love him for the unique and special person he is. (Montuschi 2000)

Community health personnel – GPs and those working in local surgeries, midwives, health visitors and mental health workers – have a key part to play in recognising the vulnerability and losses faced by couples who are going through infertility investigations and/or treatment and those who have had to use assisted conception methods in order to achieve a family.

THE TREATMENT PHASE

Specialist fertility units have one aim: that of getting women pregnant. Theirs is a technical role where the emphasis is on careful management and manipulation of a woman's monthly cycle so that her eggs (or those of a donor) should be in

BOX 12.1	*Assisted conception*

In vitro fertilisation (IVF). Following a drug regime to first close down and then artificially stimulate the woman's egg production, eggs are retrieved and placed in a dish where they are mixed with sperm from the woman's partner or a donor. Following fertilisation, the resulting embryos are assessed for quality and no more than three are returned to the woman's womb for implantation. It is the most effective treatment for women with absent, blocked or damaged fallopian tubes, plus some other conditions, including unexplained infertility. Multiple pregnancies are common.

Intracytoplasmic sperm injection (ICSI). A single sperm is taken from a semen sample or obtained surgically and is injected into the centre (cytoplasm) of an egg. This procedure is used in conjunction with IVF. This relatively new technique has made it possible for many men, who would have previously been considered totally infertile, to become genetic fathers.

Sperm donation (known as donor insemination or DI). Sperm from a donor is inserted into a woman's vagina, either next to the cervix or via intrauterine insemination into the womb, at the time of ovulation. Drugs to stimulate ovulation and/or follicle (egg) production may or may not be given. Used in instances of male infertility where ICSI is not clinically appropriate, where the couple prefer simplicity of treatment and/or consider joint parenting rather than genetic fatherhood to be more important or when ICSI is too expensive.

Egg donation. Where eggs from a donor are used instead of the eggs of the woman who wants a child. Used in conjunction with IVF. Egg donation is appropriate when a woman has gone through menopause prematurely or when pregnancy is sought late in a woman's fertile life and, despite a regular menstrual cycle, her eggs are not in good enough condition for fertilisation and/or implantation to occur. Occasionally used with donor sperm.

as ripe a condition as possible for meeting the sperm (from her husband or a donor), through carefully timed lovemaking, via a syringe and cannula (donor insemination – DI) or in a petri dish (in vitro fertilisation – IVF), with or without intracytoplasmic sperm injection (ICSI).

Some individual members of staff in fertility clinics are very aware of the emotional impact of infertility and its treatments and can be sensitive and supportive, but many couples report that clinic staff appear to be too preoccupied with procedures to acknowledge feelings. Allan (2001) notes that staff in a fertility clinic managed the emotions of patients by 'nursing the clinic and the doctor' instead of the patients.

In addition to climbing on the emotional roller-coaster that is fertility treatment, the other issue that couples have to face is how much they are able or willing to spend financially in order to have a baby. Because of the current postcode lottery of funding for fertility services, the vast majority of these treatments take place in the private sector. In December 2000, Health Secretary Alan Milburn promised that this inequity would be addressed, but funding spread thinly over the whole country may result in tighter criteria placed on eligibility for NHS treatment, most likely in the form of age limits for women entering treatment. Whatever happens, the private sector is likely to remain a key player in the provision of fertility services for the foreseeable future.

Because of this, the question, 'How much is being able to have a baby (or sometimes, 'How much is being able to have our own genetic child?') worth to us?' will remain an agonising factor in the fertility equation. The cost may include £500 to £900 required for ovarian stimulation drugs and up to £5000 for IVF with or without donated gametes or ICSI, per cycle of treatment. A GP who is sympathetic to the stress placed on infertile couples can help to lighten the load by agreeing to prescribe the necessary drugs through his or her NHS budget. Not every GP is sympathetic, however.

> The GPs are not aware of the kind of support they need to give their patients, because they don't have a clue about what you actually have to face. I've changed GPs about three times. You ask your doctor to prescribe the drugs the hospital has requested and the doctors ask what they are for. The first GP said he didn't know if he could prescribe them because I was under his care and if anything happened while I was on the drugs it would be his fault if he'd prescribed them. I said it's all in consultation with the hospital and it's not as if they're banned drugs.
> (Brian 1998:159)

The emotional impact of infertility takes on an extra dimension when the only prospect of parenthood is having a child unrelated genetically to one partner. Couples who get the news that they are going to need a sperm or egg donor to help them become parents often go through a range of responses resembling those of the grief process. And as indicated at the beginning of this chapter, men and women often react very differently. Although those who are pragmatists may want to 'get on with it', the best support professionals can give at this stage is to advise couples to take time out to talk, think and read separately and together and to put them in touch with a self-help group of people who have gone through similar experiences. Infertility can be immensely isolating. Knowing you cannot have the child of your partner and are going to need to use someone else's sperm or eggs in order to become a parent adds the dimension of having to think, what would have been only months ago, the unthinkable. The range of feelings experienced can be powerful: anger (against God, partner, the world), resentment (at partner, fertile people, medical profession), despair (at the unfairness, the inability to provide the necessary sperm or eggs), sadness (at not being able to be a genetically connected mother or father, at not being able to have a partner's child) and, more often in men than in women, a sense of being diminished as a person.

The Donor Conception Network, a national and international self-help group, can offer a safe place for both men and women to acknowledge these feelings. Unlike a visible injury or disease that attracts immediate sympathy from friends and relations and can be openly discussed, the need for gamete donation is such an intimate matter that these powerful feelings often have to be contained within the couple. Broaching the issue within wider family and friendship circles is not easy. All members of the Network have had to use, or are in the process of using, donated gametes for family creation and understand how very difficult it can be to accept that donated eggs or sperm are the only way of having a family. They are also experienced in thinking about the longer term aspects of parenting a child where there is an unknown genetic link, particularly around the issue of information sharing.

Assisted reproduction treatment may involve an extensive drug regime (for IVF) or can be relatively simple and low tech (DI). In vitro fertilisation, whether or not donated gametes are being used, is often very stressful for both the woman and her partner. The accounts in Kate Brian's book *In Pursuit of Parenthood: Real-Life Experiences of IVF* (1998) are especially valuable reading for both would-be parents and the professionals who are helping them in their attempts to get pregnant.

Under the Human Fertilisation and Embryology Act (1990), counselling has to be offered to all couples and single women undergoing assisted conception. This opportunity is not always taken up and if it is, is often felt to be cursory and inadequate. As counselling usually takes place in the clinic and often by a member of the treatment team, rather than with an independent, qualified counsellor, couples can sometimes feel inhibited about speaking freely of their concerns because they fear treatment will be withheld.

PREGNANCY

During the course of treatment many couples become very knowledgeable about hormone levels, drug doses, the nuances of investigation results and their percentage chances of having a live child. They also become extremely experienced at not being pregnant!

For the minority of those undergoing assisted conception who are lucky enough to become pregnant, fulfilment of their dreams does not always mean an end to anxiety. 'Why should things go right now? My body has done nothing but let me down. Why should I trust it to manage things properly now?' said one woman. Not all women feel this way. For many, pregnancy can be a thankful return to the 'normal' world.

TABLE 12.1	Assisted reproduction data 1998–99 (taken from Human Fertilisation and Embryology Authority Annual Report 2000)			
	Patients	Treatment cycles	Pregnancies	Children born
IVF (including ICSI)	24 306	32 292	7138	7535
Donated sperm treatments (DI + IVF with donated sperm)	5645	12 502	1736	1612
Donated egg treatments (all IVF)	1558	1702	420	451

> Prolonged infertility encourages people to anticipate loss. It convinces them that their bodies do not work right, and it heightens their awareness of what miracles conception, pregnancy and childbirth really are. Those who do become pregnant after infertility worry that something will go terribly wrong in their pregnancy. Tragically, many people do suffer miscarriages, ectopic pregnancies, and even stillbirths after infertility. Although most pregnancies are successful, even those that are medically uneventful are fraught with fear. (Glazer 1998:13)

Many women, pregnant following assisted conception, feel both fearful and abandoned as their fertility clinic cheerfully hands them over to 'normal' obstetric care. After months or years of having been carefully monitored by staff whom, despite a possibly ambivalent relationship, they have come to know well, couples suddenly find themselves alone with a pregnancy that they can hardly believe in.

ACeBabes, a charity that supports those who are using or have used assisted conception of any sort, is positive that regular contact with someone who understands the anxiety inherent in pregnancy following a long period of infertility is vital in the early weeks of pregnancy. This could be a community midwife, a GP, health visitor, practice nurse or counsellor. What counts is sensitivity to the situation, willingness to listen and acknowledge feelings and some knowledge to back up emotional support.

Many pregnant women have fantasies about the child they are carrying. For those whose baby was conceived using donated gametes, these can be particularly intense. One member of the Donor Conception Network said she had dreams of carrying a monster inside her prior to inseminations, but these disappeared when she became pregnant. For another woman, similarly alarming fantasies became more numerous as her pregnancy progressed.

STRUCTURED ANTENATAL EDUCATION

In antenatal classes, some women feel they still have little in common with other members, despite pregnancy being well established by this time. One woman quoted by Kate Brian (1998) said, 'I always used to feel everyone else was "properly" pregnant, as if my bump was somehow not quite as real as theirs'.

Surprisingly, the National Childbirth Trust, the UK's leading independent organisation supporting and educating women around childbirth, does not publish any guidance for its antenatal class teachers regarding assisted conception and its impact on parents-to-be. Childbirth educators in all settings need to be open to the signs of anxiety, beyond that experienced by most pregnant women, which might indicate that this is a very special pregnancy. Mentioning assisted conception as being much more common these days and acknowledging the range of feelings that might be associated with it, as part of an early session, could help women or couples feel less isolated and perhaps encourage them to share their experiences with class members. If the childbirth educator does suspect that a couple in the group have used assisted conception, she might want to take the opportunity to speak to them outside the session and, through listening, understand their needs better and perhaps be able to point them in the direction of a support organisation or helpful reading.

PIPPIN (Parent–Infant Partnership/Parent–Infant Network) trains midwives, health visitors and others in sensitive support and care for couples and their infant in the transition to parenthood. The Royal College of Midwives also publishes a training pack for midwives to help them meet the emotional needs of men and women as they move into parenthood.

WHO NEEDS TO KNOW?

One of the questions faced by all couples expecting an assisted conception baby is: Who needs to know? If the baby has been conceived using donated eggs or sperm, the question often feels much more complicated.

How a baby is conceived is for most people very personal information. Those who have used IVF with their own gametes (eggs or sperm) can find it helpful if close family and friends know the lengths to which they have gone to have a baby. Support from these sources can be a great comfort, but couples going through IVF often feel that they are very different from relatives, friends and workmates who seem to have conceived easily, and find it difficult to speak about what they are going through. Partly because IVF has become so common, others may assume that it is a simple, stress-free procedure, which is guaranteed to result in a pregnancy. Those going through it know only too well that this is not true. Many people, particularly women, find it helpful to be in touch with a local or national support group where they can be sure of understanding from others who have shared similar experiences.

For couples who have used donated eggs or sperm, the issues are the same but more complex. As well as the emotions generated by infertility and the treatment to get round this, couples struggle with issues to do with religious and cultural beliefs and traditions, matters of heredity, shame at not being able to be a genetic father/mother, not wanting to let their parents down and fear of stigma or censure from others. Infertile men, in particular, often find their infertility difficult to acknowledge and see themselves as diminished in some way. They are often reluctant for the use of donated sperm to be known about and many women willingly collude with their partners, allowing people to assume that the 'problem' is theirs. Unfortunately, unresolved feelings about infertility do not necessarily go away with the birth of a child conceived with donor sperm. For some men, the child is a constant reminder of their lack of fertility (so often confused in many people's minds with sexual impotency). Adult donor offspring who only learned of their origins later in life have spoken about the remoteness of fathers whom they felt (in hindsight) had never come to terms with their inability to genetically father a child (Turner & Coyle 2000). These adults have also spoken about their sense of betrayal at having been lied to; their sense of knowing there was a secret in the family and their sadness that their parents could never share their secret.

As in the past with adoption, it is only now that adult donor offspring are speaking out about their need to know more about their genetic inheritance and that their views, needs and rights are being seen as important. Slowly but surely the climate in which gamete donation is taking place in this country is changing. Women needing to use donated eggs are much more likely to share the information with family and friends. There is little stigma surrounding egg donation and many more children conceived this way are being told about their origins.

American psychologist, Susan Lewis Cooper, and social worker, Ellen Sarasohn Glazer, both work in an assisted conception clinic in Boston, USA. In their important book, *Choosing Assisted Reproduction: Social, Emotional and Ethical Considerations* (1998), they tell how their position on openness has changed over the years.

> When we entered this field, almost twenty years ago, we did not have strong opinions on this issue. Our learning and experience over the years have informed us that for ethical as well as for psychological reasons disclosure is the right approach – the one most likely to create psychologically healthy families. (p. 343)

Virtually all gamete donation in the UK is anonymous. Under the Human Fertilisation and Embryology Act 1990, sperm and egg donors recruited through licensed centres are currently guaranteed anonymity. All donor inseminations prior to the HFE Act were also anonymous but not subject to the same strict legislation. Known donors are only available through self-recruitment. In December, 2000, the government announced that it would be consulting on the question of 'origins information'. The consultation process will last for 6 months.

The key part that all general, obstetric, health visitor and mental health professionals can play is in helping men and women address the long-term issues inherent in sperm and egg donation. The parents need to understand that assisted conception is not just an issue for them as a couple but has to do with the health and welfare of a child who will become a teenager, a young adult and a parent himself. They have to consider carefully the implications of telling their child about the way in which he was conceived and, even more carefully, the implications of not telling him. Do they want to, can they live with a lie that can only become bigger and more entangled as the child gets older? Can they keep the secret through illness, separation, divorce and death? Can they manage to tell no-one else at all? Because it only takes one other person to know to let the cat out of the bag at the wrong moment. Can they really guarantee that the child will sense nothing? That they will not glance sideways at each other when relatives and friends wonder where their child's looks and talents come from?

Many parents of sperm and egg donation children worry that the child will reject them once they know the truth about their origins. The evidence from the (currently 550) families in the Donor Conception Network does not support this. In fact, one girl aged 14 has said of her father: .

> My father is 100 per cent Walter Merricks – the person who has been there since the day I was born, the man who wants me as his daughter, the man who loves me with all his heart, the man who has always been there for me and always will be. In no way would I ever consider my donor as my father, he is my genetic father but 'father' by itself sounds wrong. He gave me life and my parents great joy, but nothing else.
> (*Woman's Realm*, January 23, 2001)

For parents, the information about donor origins feels huge and unwieldy, but for well-attached, much-loved young children, it has less interest than who is coming to play or what they are having for tea. If children are told 'their story' from an early age and given small building blocks of information which match with their stage of development, then the information is integrated easily, so that when they are older they cannot remember a time when they did not know. The Donor Conception Network produces a children's picture/simple textbook, called *My Story*, suitable from age three or so, to help with this process.

The issue of 'who needs to know?' arises in pregnancy, but becomes more acute at birth and in the transition to parenthood.

BIRTH

For women who have learnt not to trust their bodies to do anything right, birth is the final opportunity for things to go wrong! Anxiety can run very high and may not be helped by doctors who want to induce a woman before term, 'just for safety's sake', because she has conceived through assisted conception. A midwife who understands and is able to acknowledge the level of anxiety, fear and unreality that may be being felt by the woman is likely to be the best birth companion, along with a supportive partner.

TRANSITION TO PARENTHOOD

Moving from being a couple to a family is acknowledged as one of life's more tricky transitions for any couple (Belsky & Kelly 1994, Cowan & Cowan 1985). Years of trying to conceive a baby do not prepare anyone for the realities of parenthood. Fantasies (and promises made to higher deities) about being the 'perfect parent' to 'perfect' children built up over the infertile months and years are challenged immediately by the exhaustion and chaos of new parenting. Parents can feel guilty for having strong negative feelings about the baby they have longed for. It is very important for midwives, health visitors, GPs, etc. to enquire carefully about how parents are feeling, rather than assume that they are unequivocally overjoyed with their new baby. Allowing negative feelings to be voiced and acknowledging them can help parents relax, stop feeling guilty and get on with enjoying their new baby and all the mixed emotions that come with early parenting.

All parents of new babies are asked, 'Who does s/he look like?' There seems to be some universal need for making connections in this way, but for parents of children conceived with the aid of donated gametes, this can be a painful moment. Their response will depend on how they have decided to handle the issue of secrecy versus openness and probably on who the enquirer is. Even the most open of parents rarely share information about their child's origins with everyone. Differentiating between secrecy and privacy, they tell those close family and friends who are likely to continue alongside them on life's journey but smile politely and agree that 'Tom looks just like his Dad' when a stranger remarks on family likenesses. Whether they choose to tell the health professionals they come into contact with may depend partly on how they feel about them. An accepting and supportive health visitor can be of enormous value to any family in the transition to parenthood but in families where the intention is not to tell the child of his origins, she can also act as an advocate, helping the parents understand the long-term implications of their decision from the perspective of the child. She can also put partners in touch with the Donor Conception Network or ACeBabes where they can share their anxieties with other parents.

In a small minority of instances, there may be a more complex transition to parenthood involving difficulties with bonding. Sensitive and supportive care in facilitating the parent–infant relationship, such as that offered by PIPPIN, can help parents acknowledge ambivalent feelings and begin to recognise their baby as a unique individual who is doing everything he can to form a relationship with them. Midwives and health visitors who know of the baby's assisted conception should be aware of the small risk of bonding difficulties and be prepared to seek specialist help if needed. It is helpful if one member of a community health team is knowledgeable about the impact of infertility and its treatments on pregnancy, birth and beyond, so that she or he can be a resource for colleagues.

LONGER TERM ISSUES

Parenting

Those who have had to struggle so hard to have their children sometimes find the normal 'letting go' processes – starting nursery and school, wanting to be with friends rather than parents, adolescence – hard to bear, as these transitions can rekindle earlier feelings of loss. They also have to discover that love is not enough. Their child, like any other, needs a balance of nurture and guidance/teaching for them to feel secure and to be able to develop friendships and learn.

Professionals, including teachers, who understand about the anxieties felt by many parents of children conceived through assisted conception can be of great value in helping parents acknowledge their feelings and in providing information about child development and appropriate parental responses. They can give permission to a parent to behave 'normally' rather than feeling she cannot possibly say 'No' to such a special child.

Parents whose children were conceived with donated gametes are likely to feel more secure about the relationship with their children as time passes and the family progresses and develops like any other. They will, however, need to continually address the 'need to know' issue as children move through school, have medical examinations, etc. They will also need to be alive to their children's changing awareness of, and interest in, their origins. The Donor Conception Network can help with all these matters.

How parents feel themselves

ACeBabes members are clear that despite having achieved pregnancy and the longed-for state of parenthood, they do not feel the same as other parents. At a meeting in October 2000, members of the Derby group spoke movingly about how they and their partners felt changed as people because of the emotional turmoil they had been through. On the one hand they felt they had matured and become more understanding of others and on the other, believed they had become more cynical. Families where infertility has been resolved fairly quickly, even if donated gametes have been used, are likely to feel they have more in common with other parents.

ASSISTED CONCEPTION WITHOUT INFERTILITY

Not only heterosexual couples will seek to use assisted conception methods. Lesbian couples have long used sperm donated by a male friend as a way of bringing a child into their relationship and single (usually heterosexual) women are increasingly using donated sperm to have a baby, in the absence of a life partner with whom to conceive a child. Professionals who come into contact with women who have achieved pregnancy this way may have strong feelings about family creation outside a heterosexual relationship. It will be important for them to be able to acknowledge their personal values and beliefs but to keep an open mind as they support a new parent setting out to create the best life possible for her child. The role of the health visitor in supporting lesbian couples and their children is set out in Salmon & Hall (1999).

KEY POINTS

- *Prolonged* infertility is a challenging and life-changing experience for both men and women.
- Professionals who come into contact with couples experiencing infertility or parenting following infertility treatment need to be able to reflect on their own feelings about infertility and assisted conception methods.
- In vitro fertilisation, although now commonplace, remains an invasive, physically and emotionally stressful, often very expensive and not highly successful procedure.
- Feelings of loss, in some form or other, may remain, even when pregnancy is achieved and a healthy child born.
- Families where members have been created with the help of assisted conception are both different from and just like any other family.
- Honesty with children about their origins, particularly when donated eggs, embryo or sperm have aided conception, is the best option for long-term happy and healthy family relationships.

REFERENCES

Allan HT 2001 Nursing the clinic and managing emotions in a fertility unit: findings from an ethnographic study. Human Fertility 4 (1): 18–23

Belsky J, Kelly J 1994 The transition to parenthood: how a first child changes a marriage. Vermilion, London

Brian K 1998 In pursuit of parenthood: real-life experiences of IVF. Bloomsbury, London

Cooper SL, Glazer ES 1998 Choosing assisted reproduction: social, emotional and ethical considerations. Perspectives Press, Indianapolis, USA

Cowan CP, Cowan PA 1985 Transitions to parenthood, his, hers and theirs. Journal of Family Issues 6 (4):451–481

Glazer ES 1998 The long-awaited stork: a guide to parenting after infertility. Jossey-Bass, San Francisco

Johnston PI 1994 Taking charge of infertility. Perspectives Press, Indianapolis, USA

Montuschi O 2000 Parenting children conceived using donated eggs or sperm: is it different? DC Network News, Newsletter No. 15, 3–4

Salmon D, Hall C 1999 Working with lesbian mothers: their healthcare experiences. Community Practitioner 72 (12): 396–397

Turner AJ, Coyle A 2000 What does it mean to be a donor offspring? Human Reproduction 15 (9):2041–2051

FURTHER READING

One or two of these books are American, as are some of the references. Do not let this put you off – they are excellent, despite the differences in law and regulations regarding assisted conception and adoption. All books, except *My Story*, can be obtained from Internet book sites, e.g. Amazon.co.uk

Bernstein AC 1994 Flight of the stork: what children think (and when) about sex and family building. Perspectives Press, Indianapolis, USA

Blyth E 1995 Infertility and assisted conception: practice issues for counsellors. British Association of Social Workers, Birmingham

Blyth E, Crawshaw M, Speirs J (eds) 1998 Truth and the child 10 years on: information exchange in donor assisted conception. British Association of Social Workers, Birmingham

Elton B 1999 Inconceivable (also the film version *Maybe Baby*). Black Swan, London

Infertility Research Trust 1991 My story. A book about family building through DI, for 3–6 year olds. Available from the Donor Conception Network (see below).

McWhinnie A 2001 Should offspring from donated gametes continue to be denied knowledge of their origins and antecedents? Human Reproduction 16(5): 807–817

Montuschi O, Merricks W 2000 Why children need to know. Available from Progress Education Trust, 140 Gray's Inn Road, London WC1X 8AX
Tel: 020 7278 7870
Fax: 020 7278 7862
Website: www.progress.org.uk

Schnitter JT 1995 Let me explain: a story about donor insemination (for 7 to 12 year olds). Perspectives Press, Indianapolis, USA

Scott M 2000 Genes, anonymity and donor conception. Progress in Reproduction 4 (3): 6–7

Vercollone C, Moss H, Moss R 1997 Helping the Stork: the choices and challenges of donor insemination. McMillan, London

RESOURCES

Transition to Parenting
Royal College of Midwives, 15 Mansfield Street, London W1M 0BE
Tel: 020 7312 3535
Fax: 020 7312 3536
Training pack consisting of five A4 booklets. Includes excellent chapters on transition to motherhood and fatherhood and the changing social context of parenting. Although they do not mention the specific issues of assisted reproduction, anyone following the practice recommended in these booklets would be likely to be sensitive to the emotional and support needs of this group of parents.

Useful organisations

Donor Conception Network, PO Box 265, Sheffield S3 7YX
Tel/fax: 0208 245 4369
Email: dcnetwork@appleonline.net
Website: www.dcnetwork.org
Parent-led charity which offers emotional and social support/information and guidance to anyone using donated gametes for family creation and those who are adult offspring. Professionals are welcome as associate members.

AceBabes, c/o Doriver Lilley, 8 Yarwell Close, Derwent Heights, Derby DE21 4SW
Tel: 01332 832558 or 0115 987 9266
Email: enquiries@acebabes.co.uk
Website: www.acebabes.co.uk
This charity was set up to meet the support and information needs of parents who have used assisted conception and those currently going through treatment (with or without donated gametes).

CHILD, Charter House, 43 St Leonards Road, Bexhill on Sea, East Sussex TN40 1JA
Tel: 01424 732361
Fax: 01424 731858
Email: office@child.org.uk
Website: www.child.org.uk
For advice, support and information regarding fertility clinics, treatments and local fertility support groups.

Human Fertilisation and Embryology Authority, 30 Artillery Lane, London
E1 7LS
Tel: 020 7377 5077
Fax: 020 7377 1871
Website: www.hfea.gov.uk
The statutory regulatory body for assisted reproductive technology publishes an annual report and accounts and two guides to assisted reproduction clinics: The Patients' Guide to DI and The Patients' Guide to IVF Clinics.

PIPPIN (Parent–Infant Partnership/Parent–Infant Network), Catherine Joyce, Assistant Director, Projects, Services and Training, 34 Chandlers Road, St Albans, Herts AL4 9RS
Tel: 01727 840 540
Fax: 01727 848 444
Email: catherine@pippin.org.uk
Website: www.pippin.org.uk
Provides training in sensitive facilitation of the parent–infant relationship, to professionals and others who work with parents in the transition to parenthood.

13 Evaluating parenting education

Mary Nolan

INTRODUCTION

It is notoriously difficult to evaluate an educational intervention. Evaluating how effective a drug is in the treatment of some illness lends itself to a scientific approach. Patients can be treated as 'cases', each having in common the symptoms of the particular disease. The drug can be administered in controlled doses on a predetermined number of occasions. Outcome measures can be clearly defined. None of this is true of education where each learner brings to the educational encounter an entirely different personal history, different learning needs and different attitudes towards learning.

Lumley & Brown's seminal study (1993) of attenders and non-attenders at antenatal classes concluded that attendance at classes was not associated with any differences in birth events, women's satisfaction with the care they received or with their emotional well-being after giving birth. A damning indictment, you might think, and enough to keep women away from classes and childbirth educators from continuing their work. But were the right outcomes identified? How multifaceted is 'emotional well-being' and how utterly impossible to measure all of those facets! Might it be that the impact of classes cannot be detected immediately after the birth, but becomes apparent months or even years later? Gould (1986) comments that the changes brought about by health education are subtle, 'may not become apparent for years and may never be unequivocally related to intervention' (p. 59).

WHY EVALUATE?

If the difficulties are so enormous in evaluating education, why bother? The answer is that there is an ethical obligation to evaluate any intervention to ensure that there are no detrimental effects on the people exposed to it. You have an obligation to evaluate because your time is precious and your skills should be put to the best use possible and because your clients' time is equally precious and they deserve the best and most appropriate service which you can provide for them. In an era of cost consciousness, there is a need to ensure that health professionals' salaries represent value for money in terms of the way in which time is spent with clients.

Tones & Tilford (1996) consider that evaluation can be used for a range of purposes.

- To provide feedback to activities and projects.
- For dissemination to others.

■ For developing theory about activities and contexts studied.
■ For accounting purposes – assessing the worth in terms of effectiveness, efficiency and equity. (p. 50)

The purpose of this book has been to assist health professionals in moving away from theories of education (generally well covered in pre-registration and postregistration courses) to their implementation in practice (generally less well covered in such courses). This chapter looks at practical ways in which you can evaluate the education you are providing for parents and find the evidence to present to managers that what you are doing is effective.

THE REFLECTIVE PRACTITIONER

Adey & Shayer (1994) remind professionals that good practitioners have internalised theories and structures, so allowing them to modify practice in the light of feedback. It is therefore necessary to identify a structure that will enable you to obtain high-quality feedback and subsequently to use the feedback to change your practice. Such theories abound and the one that is best is the one that is most useful to you. 'Reflection-on-action' (Schon 1983) allows you to consider in a structured way what happened during the educational encounter after it is over and to determine whether what you did enabled you to provide the richest possible learning opportunities for the parents. This is not to forget the importance of 'reflection-*in*-action' when the educator, constantly aware of the aims of the course, its content, the parents' needs, the parents' response to the material being presented and the importance of good time management, adjusts her teaching approaches almost from minute to minute in order to keep all these balls in the air.

Reflective practice is often described as a cycle (Atkins & Murphy 1996, Bond et al 1985, Kolb 1984) and it needs to be thought of as a dynamic *process*, a thoughtful and restless engagement with our practice as educators which ensures that the service we offer to parents improves continuously. The cycle might run through planning a class or course, executing it, obtaining feedback from a variety of sources (more about how to do this later) and then evaluating and analysing the feedback.

Feedback enables us to identify:

■ the strengths of the course/educational encounter
■ the weaknesses
■ the threats (either internal or external) that hampered or might hamper the effectiveness of the course
■ the opportunities for future work with parents.

We can then make plans to build on the strengths of the course, rectify the weaknesses, minimise the threats and seize the opportunities.

A reflective approach to evaluation might involve analysing in a very personal way your engagement with the parent or parents whom you were educating. The following ideas are based on Johns' structured reflection (1998). Start by describing to yourself (or, better still, to a colleague) the class you led or your encounter with the parents. Then ask yourself some cue questions.

| BOX 13.1 | *Structured reflection* |

- What was I trying to achieve in the class/interview/meeting with the parents?
- How were the parents feeling?
- How do I know they were feeling like that?
- How did I feel in the situation?
- What internal and external factors influenced the way I related to the parents?
  Internal factors, e.g.
  - whether my mind was concentrated on the task in hand or distracted by other thoughts
  - how I was feeling emotionally
  - whether I was well or feeling ill or hungry or cold
  - whether I liked the parents with whom I was working
  - whether the topic was one that had a personal resonance for me.
    External factors, e.g.
  - whether the environment was appropriate for this encounter
  - whether I was interrupted during my meeting with the parents
  - whether I was in a rush to get away or the parents were
  - whether I was being observed.
- Did my approach to the parents match with my beliefs? Or did I behave in incongruent ways? Why?
- How does the experience of this class or meeting connect with previous similar experience I have had?
- Could I handle this situation better in future? How?
- What would be the consequences of acting differently? For myself? For the parents?
- How do I feel NOW about the class/meeting?

It is much easier to work through these questions in a truly challenging way if you have someone to prompt your ideas, ask you to clarify what you have said and prevent you from sliding off the topic in hand. So choose a colleague with good listening and reflecting skills to work with you.

EVALUATING PRACTICAL ARRANGEMENTS

Before you look at the content of the classes you have led, the teaching approaches that you used and how much learning parents either did or did not achieve, you need to look at whether the practical arrangements went well. These are the details which attract parents to classes and keep them coming. If the parents don't attend in the first place, you can't teach them anything!

- *Timing* – did the day of the week and the times of the classes enable as many parents as possible to attend?
- *Your convenience* – did the course fit in with the rest of your work/private commitments? Can you sustain it in the long term?

- *Venue* – was the venue easily accessible for the parents who wished to attend? How many had to catch one bus? Two buses? How many had to get a lift? Or borrow the car? How many could walk to the venue? Were facilities appropriate for parents with mobility difficulties? Or hearing difficulties, etc.?

- *Comfort* – what were the toilet facilities like? Were there refreshments available? Was the room warm/cool according to season? Were the chairs comfortable? Was there enough space for small group work to be carried out in privacy?

- How many parents attended individual classes of the course? How many came to every class? What was the drop-out rate? At what stage in the course did people drop out?

- *Cost* – how much did it cost you to put on this course? How much did it cost parents to attend?

- *Advertising* – did your advertising reach the people it was intended to reach? What were the most successful sources of advertising?

There are a variety of ways of getting answers to these questions. If your group of parents is comfortable with pen and paper, you could ask them to fill in a questionnaire. If the parents are not, you could talk to them as a group or individually, asking for some feedback. If there seems to be a great deal of dissatisfaction with the practical arrangements for the course, you could ask a couple of parents to work with you to identify what would be better.

You will also want to evaluate the effectiveness of the learning opportunities you provided and this applies to running courses or to seeing parents on an individual basis in a health clinic or for a one-to-one session to address a particular parenting issue.

EVALUATING THE LEARNING ACHIEVED: USING AIMS AND LEARNING OUTCOMES

It may not be possible to evaluate an educational intervention in such a way that its impact can be entirely understood or quantified in some way. This does not mean that there are no facets of the intervention that can be quite rigorously evaluated or that less tangible facets cannot be evaluated to some extent. In order to satisfy supervisors and managers that time and money are being well spent (not to mention your own need to know that what you are doing is useful), you have to devise some means of evaluating the educational enterprise in which you have engaged with the parents.

Whether you are teaching a group or working with a parent or a family on an individual basis, it is essential to have clearly formulated what it is you are hoping that your clients will learn and what it is that they are hoping to learn. Some of these things will be difficult to evaluate, but some will be quite straightforward.

It is a very useful exercise to start to formulate aims and learning outcomes for any educational encounter that you engage in with parents. Aims are broad statements about what you hope to achieve. They are very difficult to measure in 'scientific' terms but you can spot indications that progress is being made with them. Learning outcomes are specific, limited and eminently measurable. So, for example, if you are working with a group of parents of preschool children, you might formulate your aims thus.

- To boost parents' confidence in their instinctive parenting skills.
- To raise parents' awareness of their attitudes towards parenting and of the roots of those attitudes.
- To encourage parents to help each other in dealing with problems with their children.

Your learning outcomes will focus on the learning that can (or might) be seen to have been achieved and might be phrased thus.

By the end of this parenting course, the parents will be able to:

- play with their children in a variety of ways and understand the value of playing
- describe and put into practice two strategies for coping with toddler tantrums
- describe the kind of language that undermines small children's confidence and the kind that fosters their self-esteem
- talk about the impact their own childhood experiences have had on their approach to parenting
- list three professionals/organisations to which they can turn for help.

Learning outcomes do not lend themselves to fudging. You apply them to every member of your group and ask whether each person achieved each outcome. If you feel that some of the parents did not, ask yourself how you could improve the course so that next time, a higher proportion of the group achieves all the outcomes.

EVALUATING COGNITIVE AND PSYCHOMOTOR LEARNING

Education operates in three domains, the cognitive, the affective and the practical. The cognitive, which is to do with acquiring knowledge and understanding, can be evaluated using learning outcomes as a tool. It is not too difficult to find out whether people have gained knowledge (although the acquisition of knowledge does not necessarily imply that they will apply that knowledge either in the best way possible or at all). The practical domain can also be tested. You can ask people to demonstrate a skill (although, once again, you cannot be sure that people will continue to practise skills they have acquired). Although we would hope that education leads to changes in lifestyle and to a better quality of life for learners, it is difficult to gather the evidence to prove that this is the case. This issue will be discussed later in the chapter.

Factual knowledge is comparatively easy to test, although it is more difficult to be sure that it is retained in the longer term.

Most students seem to have inherited incredibly powerful forgetting mechanisms that can be triggered by such stimuli as air, soil or water. It is probably more sensible for instructors to think of students as wide-gauge sieves through which acquired knowledge runs out at blinding speed. (Popham 1988:301)

Formulating learning outcomes should help you feel confident that information and skills have been transmitted, at least in the short term; you will need to check that they have been retained when you next see the parents. Being clear about learning outcomes is particularly useful when the knowledge and understanding that parents need are essential for their child's health and emotional well-being. For example, you might visit a family which includes a child with cystic fibrosis and you have to ensure that the child is brought for regular physiotherapy. What do the parents need to know? Your learning outcomes might be as follows.

By the end of my visit, the parents will be able to:

- explain why regular physiotherapy is important for their child
- say when and where the child's next appointment with the physiotherapist is
- rearrange the appointment if they are unable to keep it
- demonstrate a daily routine of physiotherapy that they will carry out with their child.

You can then think about how you are going to get this information across in such a way that the parents' sense of responsibility for the welfare of their child is not undermined and their feeling that they are in control of their own lives is safeguarded (your aims). You will probably want the parents to tell you the details of their appointment and how they are going to get to the clinic or hospital. You will want to be sure that the way in which they describe their child's condition and his needs represent an accurate understanding of cystic fibrosis. You will listen to what they have to say about their dealings with the hospital to evaluate whether they know how to work 'the system'. In these ways, you can check whether the necessary learning has been achieved.

This is a simple example but my intention is to make the point that formulating in your own mind, or even on paper, what the essence of the educational encounter is enables you to feel confident that the essential facts and skills have been achieved by parents.

EVALUATING AFFECTIVE LEARNING

Learning in the affective domain is much the most difficult to measure. How can you assess whether people's attitudes have changed or undergone modification? How can you know that prejudices have been erased? How can you be sure that people have become more able to reflect on their feelings and behaviour and to use their self-evaluation to change the way in which they approach the challenges facing them in their lives? In summary, how do you know that your clients have achieved increased adulthood and greater autonomy?

It is easy to assume that changes must be taking place in our clients as a result of our carefully thought-through educational interventions. And when challenged to define or demonstrate those changes, to retort that they are subtle, not readily on display and do not lend themselves to quantification. Yet not to attempt to assess whether any change in people's attitudes has taken place is surely to abrogate responsibility for the outcome of our teaching. After all, the changes that have taken place in the affective domain might not be positive ones. Harm might have been done that needs to be rectified before the parents leave the remit of our care.

A series of classes can incorporate a number of opportunities for educators to assess the trajectory of parents' learning in the affective domain. Role play is a particularly useful tool. Although people are often unwilling to participate, once they do it can be hard to stop them developing the scenario ad infinitum! Rather like putting on a mask, role play can provide a safe way of being yourself yet being someone other who does not have to take responsibility for words and actions. You might want to describe a scenario where the 'mother' and 'father' have to deal with their 16-year-old 'daughter' who has returned home at midday the day after she went to a night club, promising to be back by one in the morning. If you set this role play up towards the end of your course, you might get some clues as to how much your clients have learned about maintaining a balance between understanding their child's need for autonomy and their own need to know that she is safe.

You might set up a role play where the mother is out shopping with a toddler whose (quite normal) behaviour is criticised by another shopper. Can you tell by observing the role play what your clients have learned about assertiveness?

Or you might enact a scene where a father takes his son to the hospital for an appointment with a specialist and needs to obtain information about his child's condition and treatment from a not very forthcoming doctor. Does the man playing the father know the questions to ask and how to ask them?

If role play is not for you (or your clients), you could present the group with a scenario written down on card for them to discuss in twos and threes (for one example, see Activity 13.1).

As the group leader, your task is not simply to provide first-rate learning opportunities for the parents but to observe them, stand in their shoes, read between the lines of their conversation and try and understand where they are coming from. You can gain a great deal of information about how people are feeling from:

- their body language (open? receptive? closed? guarded?)
- the questions they ask
- their level of contribution to the discussion
- their engagement with the rest of the group

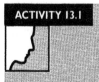

ACTIVITY 13.1

JOSHUA HATES SCHOOL

Joshua is 7 years old. He is always in trouble at school, generally for pushing other children in the playground, elbowing his way to the front of the dinner queue and not paying attention in class. His mother has been invited to speak to the head teacher on three occasions. She has two other small children at home and her partner works long hours and night shifts and is able to offer very little help. How might the mother handle this situation?

- the way in which they make links between what is being discussed and their own experiences
- the statements they make about doing things differently/seeking more information/planning to talk to their partner, mother-in-law, GP, social worker, health visitor . . .

You might design a questionnaire to test people's attitudes. This is, of course, not as easy as it sounds. If you want in-depth guidance, consult Oppenheim (1992). People often fill in questionnaires according to what they think are the 'right' answers, rather than according to what they really think. You are more likely to find out their real views if they fill in the questionnaire anonymously. You might choose to use the same questionnaire at the beginning and at the end of your course to see whether any changes in the parents' approach to key situations have occurred (see Activity 13.2).

ACTIVITY 13.2

Some parents would say that a slap is the right way of dealing with a child who is doing something dangerous. What do you think?

Agree   ☐
Disagree   ☐
Not sure   ☐

Hayley's 14-year-old daughter Emma tells her that she has slept with a man in his 30s because he said it was best for her to have her first experience of sex with an older man. Who do you think Hayley should talk to?

The man   ☐
Emma's GP   ☐
The police   ☐
Emma's head teacher   ☐
Emma's father   ☐
No-one unless Emma agrees ☐

FEEDBACK FROM COLLEAGUES

You can measure your own performance against your aims and learning outcomes, as described above. However, no matter how honest you are in challenging yourself as to whether you achieved what you, and the parents, hoped to achieve, it is very difficult to see yourself as others see and hear you. This is why it is absolutely invaluable to ask a colleague to observe you teaching a class, leading a group or interviewing a parent. Choose a colleague:

- whose skills in teaching and communicating you admire
- who listens well
- who is non-judgemental but clear and straightforward in what she says
- who will not be hampered by her own baggage (personal or professional) in giving you feedback.

You might like to agree a checklist of areas which your colleague will comment on, such as the following.

- *Language* – was it always appropriate for the parent or group; was it sensitive, non-judgemental?
- *Listening skills* – were you able to hear what parents were saying to you about the issues that really matter to them; can you cope with silences which occur while people sort out their ideas?
- *Group skills* – were you able to involve every member of the group as much as they wanted to be involved and help the group to get to know each other and listen to each other?
- *Valuing people's experiences* – did you help people to talk about their experiences and build on them?
- *Variety of teaching methods* – did you cater for parents who are visual learners, those who are auditory learners and those who are kinaesthetic learners?
- *Handling your own prejudices* – did you always present issues in a balanced manner, betraying no personal prejudices?
- *Key issues* – were you able to help parents identify and discuss what were the key issues for them?
- *Knowledge base* – is the information that you gave to parents accurate and up to date?
- *Teaching women/men* – if you are a male educator, did you enable the women to participate as fully as the men? Did you help them identify their key issues? If you are a female educator, did you enable the men to participate as fully as the women and help them identify their key issues?
- *Visual aids/teaching aids* – were these of a high quality, attractive and relevant? Did you allow the parents to handle them so that they had 'ownership' of the materials of their own learning?
- *Planning* – was the class planned so as to enable parents to achieve the maximum amount of learning?
- *Time management* – was the pace of the class fast enough to maintain everyone's interest, while being sufficiently relaxed to enable people to explore their concerns?
- *Environment* – had you tried to make the environment in which the class/interview was held as pleasant as possible to enhance learning?

Clearly, not all of these questions will be relevant in every educational situation. The appropriate questions to focus on will depend on whether your colleague is observing you helping a mother with learning difficulties understand how to provide a stimulating environment for her preschool children or whether you are leading an antenatal class for eight couples or facilitating a discussion group for parents of teenagers. Choose the questions that are relevant and ask your colleague to give you feedback that is as detailed and honest as possible. Discuss with her the way forward – what improvements could you make in order to be more effective as an educator? Ask if you can observe her in a similar situation so that you can learn from her. Watching other people working with parents is an extremely useful way of evaluating your own skills. It gives you a yardstick against which to measure what you are doing yourself and how much you are achieving. You will also get lots of useful ideas for new ways of working with parents.

Instead of choosing a colleague to observe you, you might choose a parent whom you know or have worked with. The parent might use a different kind of language to give you feedback from that which your colleague would use, but if both are good observers, the underlying themes that they pick out will be the same.

HANDLING FEEDBACK

It is very human to look through a pile of evaluation forms which parents have completed at the end of their parenting course and see only the negative things that they have written. The comments regarding what was not so good about the course leap off the page, while the many complimentary remarks are skimmed over. Read through the forms once and then come back to them later. You will be able to take a more balanced view when the initial nervousness about reading them has worn off.

Look at the ratio of negative to positive comments – you will probably find that the latter far outweigh the former. Ignore the 'one-off' comments such as 'Rubbish!' and 'Totally brilliant' and look closely at the comments that demonstrate a real effort on the part of the parent to tell you what he or she enjoyed about the course and found helpful and what was not of relevance. Identify themes; if a lot of people say that they did not find the session on handling toddler tantrums helpful, you need to have another look at how you are covering that issue. If a lot of people say positive things about the discussion on how to talk about sex to preadolescent children, that discussion obviously went well and should be retained for the next course.

If a parent or colleague has observed you working with parents either on an individual basis or in a group, make sure that you ask them to summarise their thoughts under three headings: what was good about your work, what was not so good, and how they think you might improve. Evaluation should never be static – it should leave you feeling energised and eager to move forwards in your practice.

You might feel in the middle of a class or course that things are not going well. Stop and ask the parents to help you. Ask them if they are learning what they hoped to learn and, if not, what changes are required. Do not accept criticism from people if they cannot suggest how the service could be improved. It is easy to criticise, but to reflect on the educational encounter in a way that leads the educator forward demands a truly mature and insightful intelligence.

LONG-TERM FEEDBACK

Even when parents no longer come directly within the remit of your care, it is likely that you will hear about how they are getting on from other colleagues. What happens to them after they move on cannot be laid directly at your door but you could certainly reflect on their future careers in the light of the educational encounters that you had with them. If you hear of parents continuing to attend a parenting group or taking up other educational opportunities or becoming involved in setting up a parenting support group themselves, this would suggest that the opportunity you provided for them to learn from others and gain support from their peers was appreciated and has been acted upon. It would be interesting to monitor how often parents who have attended a parenting course consult their GPs about either their own or their children's minor physical and mental health problems in the year after attending. Does this say something about how you helped them to grow in confidence as parents and to gain skills for handling the day-to-day problems that arise with children and young people? You could look at the extent of Social Services involvement with parents whom you have taught. Have parents managed to cope on their own or have they had to rely on the support of statutory agencies?

These are very rough measures of the effectiveness of your educational intervention because so many other factors will influence the future life courses of the parents with whom you have come into contact. Nevertheless, education attempts to nurture problem-solving skills in adult learners and a legitimate measure of its success in doing this is the extent to which parents do solve their own problems, either on their own or supported by other parents.

THE POLITICAL AGENDA

Cowan (1997) states that: 'Deep learning is learning that will actually result in different behaviour' (p. 159).

It is not always possible to know whether the educational encounter with parents will change their parenting practice in either the short or the long term. However, there is no harm in keeping a political agenda in mind when you act as an educator. Education is about critical consciousness raising. Enkin et al (1995), writing about antenatal parenting classes, describe an empowerment model of health education.

> The full impact of childbirth education cannot be assessed solely by its effect on the individual woman giving birth, for there may be indirect effects that engender significant changes in the ambience in which all women give birth. Once a critical mass of mothers becomes aware of the fact that options are available to them, major changes in obstetrical practice may ensue. (p. 20)

The same is true of any other kind of parenting education. What we are hoping for is that as parents' understanding of the task of parenting is enhanced and the impact of environmental, social, financial and personal stressors on parents and their children is better appreciated, parents will act at community and national levels through the voting system to demand better conditions under which to carry on the job of parenting. Tones & Tilford (1996) remind us how education moves from the micro level to the macro (Fig. 13.1), just as the ripples from a stone dropped into the middle of a pond will eventually reach its outermost limits.

| FIGURE 13.1 | *Levels of education (based on Tones & Tilford 1996)* |

Macro

National policy level

Strategic level

Mass media, community development, social action

Settings

Schools, workplace, primary care, the home

Methods

One to one, support groups, discussion groups, classes, role play, games, life skills

Resources

Cooperation with voluntary bodies, videos, leaflets, Internet, posters, etc.

Micro

CONCLUSION

This book has been about what kind of education parents need, first as adult learners and second as individual parents with particular needs, and about how that education might most effectively be delivered. The authors have provided a host of practical ideas to help you 'educate' (and we have accepted a very broad definition of that word, which originally meant simply 'leading out') parents, in whatever circumstances you meet them. You are bound to come across intractable situations where the quality of parenting is poor and likely to remain so because of the desperate circumstances in which families find themselves. Yet empowering parents to ask questions, to identify and access resources to help them cope, to seek further educational opportunities, to group together with other parents to lobby for change in their locality – all these are the building blocks upon which the edifice of change is built. Ultimately, we are engaged in education for citizenship and 'progress towards maximal versions of citizenship, incorporating competence and capability for action and social contribution' (Evans 1998: 134).

The quality of parenting is fundamental to the quality of any society anywhere in the world. Never has parenting been under so much pressure as it is at present in the affluent world. Education for parenting has the potential to change the ways in which we relate to each other, affecting our own and our children's happiness. The opportunity to be engaged in this initiative is a privilege and we should certainly embrace it with some of the revolutionary spirit of Paulo Freire (1972).

To affirm that men and women are persons and as persons should be free, and yet to do nothing tangible to make this affirmation a reality, is a farce. (p. 25)

- There is an ethical obligation to evaluate any educational or support intervention to ensure that the people exposed to it experience no adverse effects.

- It is important to identify a structure to obtain high-quality feedback which can then be used to improve practice.

- As well as assessing how much knowledge clients have acquired, it is important to look at whether changes in attitude have taken place as a result of the educational initiative.

- A legitimate measure of the success of parenting education is the extent to which parents can solve their own problems, either on their own or supported by other parents.

- As parents gain more insight into the impact of environmental, social, financial and personal stressors on them and their children, they may choose to act at the level of their community and at national level through the voting system to demand better conditions under which to carry on the job of parenting.

REFERENCES

Adey P, Shayer M 1994 Really raising standards. Routledge, London

Atkins S, Murphy K 1996 Reflective practice. Continuing Education in Nursing 329: 27–31

Boud D, Keogh R, Walker D (eds) 1985 Reflection: turning experience into learning. Kogan Page, London

Cowan L 1997 What you need to know about continuing your education – portfolios, profiles, diplomas, degrees. MIDIRS 2(2): 156–159

Enkin M, Keirse MJNC, Renfrew M, Neilson J 1995 A guide to effective care in pregnancy and childbirth, 2nd edn. Oxford University Press, Oxford

Evans KM 1998 Shaping futures: learning for competence and citizenship. Ashgate, Aldershot

Freire P 1972 Pedagogy of the oppressed (trans. Ramos MB). Herder and Herder, New York

Gould D 1986 Locally organised antenatal classes and their effectiveness. Nursing Times 82(45): 59–61

Johns C (ed) 1998 Transforming nursing through reflective practice. Blackwell Science, Oxford

Kolb D 1984 Experiential learning. Prentice Hall, Englewood Cliffs, New Jersey

Lumley J, Brown S 1993 Attenders and nonattenders at childbirth education classes in Australia: how do they and their births differ? Birth 20 (3): 123–130

Oppenheim AN 1992 Questionnaire design, interviewing and attitude measurement. Pinter, London

Popham WJ 1988 Educational evaluation. Prentice Hall, Englewood Cliffs, New Jersey

Schon D 1983 The reflective practitioner: how professionals think in action. Basic Books, New York

Tones K, Tilford S 1996 Health education: effectiveness, efficiency and equity, 2nd edn. Chapman and Hall, London

Index

Printed and bound by CPI Group (UK) Ltd, Croydon, CR0 4YY

03/10/2024

01040364-0004